SOLVING THE GLUTEN PUZZLE

DISCOVERING GLUTEN SENSITIVITY AND EMBRACING THE GLUTEN-FREE LIFESTYLE

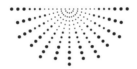

SUSAN U. NEAL RN, MBA, MHS

CHRISTIAN INDIE PUBLISHING

Editor: Janis Whipple

Cover Design: Brooke Neal

Printed in the United States of America

ISBN: 978-1-7336443-1-0

Medical Disclaimer: This book offers health and nutritional information, which is for educational purposes only. The information provided in this book is designed to help individuals make informed decisions about their health; it is intended to supplement, not replace, the professional medical advice, diagnosis, or treatment of health conditions from a trained medical professional. Please consult your physician or healthcare provider before beginning or changing any health or eating habits to make sure that it is appropriate for you. If you have any concerns or questions about your health, you should always ask a physician or other healthcare provider. Please do not disregard, avoid, or delay obtaining medical or health-related advice from your healthcare professional because of something you may have read in this book. The author and publisher assume no responsibility for any injury that may result from changing your health or eating habits.

Disclaimer and Terms of Use: Every effort has been made to ensure the information in this book is accurate and complete. However, the author and publisher do not warrant the accuracy or completeness of the material, text, and graphics contained in this book. The author and publisher do not hold any responsibility for errors, omissions, or contrary interpretation of the subject matter contained herein. This book is presented for motivational, educational, and informational purposes only. This book is sold with the understanding that the author and publisher are not engaged in rendering medical, legal, or other professional advice or services. Neither the publisher nor the author shall be liable for damages arising herein.

*Thank you
to the individuals willing to share
their gluten-related stories
so others could benefit.*

TABLE OF CONTENTS

A GIFT FOR YOU

I am excited you decided to take this journey of health and wellness. To help you determine if you are intolerant to gluten, I created a gluten quiz. To receive the quiz, go to SusanUNeal.com/GlutenQuiz.

Join my Facebook group, Facebook.com/7 Steps to Get Off Sugar, Carbs, and Gluten where I am available to answer your questions and provide you with encouragement and support you may need.

I created the Healthy Living Blog to provide you with helpful articles, menus, recipes, and lifestyle tips. You can subscribe to it at SusanUNeal.com/Healthy-Living-Blog.

I created the Facebook page Healthy Living Series to keep you up-to-date with relevant information about a healthy lifestyle. Check out and click the like button at Facebook.com/HealthyLivingSeries.

If you need additional support making this lifestyle change, purchase my course, 7 Steps to Reclaim Your Health and Optimal Weight (https://susanuneal.com/courses/7-steps-to-get-off-sugar-and-carbs-course). In this course I walk you through all the material covered in my Healthy Living Series. I help you change your eating habits once and for all.

If you want to find out if you suffer from gluten intolerance, take the Gluten Quiz at GlutenIntoleranceQuiz.com.

PREFACE

Have you experienced health issues that doctors could not cure or diagnose? This book can help you determine whether your health problems are connected to a gluten-related disorder. As a registered nurse with a master's degree in health science, I can help you determine if you are gluten sensitive and teach you what I learned from personal experience with a gluten diagnosis. As a child I was allergic to wheat; as an adult I suffer from wheat sensitivity. Recently we discovered my daughter is gluten sensitive. However, it took over a decade to diagnose her.

Unfortunately, gluten-related conditions are no longer rare; scientists estimate 10 percent of the population is affected by one.[1] If by reading this book you discover that gluten harms your body, don't be discouraged because you will also learn how to embrace the gluten-free lifestyle so you can feel well again.

Join me and discover if sensitivity to gluten is the answer to your health challenges.

Susan U. Neal

INTRODUCTION

Martin's Story

At sixty-three Martin experienced more than the usual amount of health issues for a man his age. Though he had good days and bad, on the bad days, the symptoms were debilitating, and always the same. His chest tightened as if a belt squeezed his upper body. Next, needle-prick sensations moved down his lower body as he expelled several firm bowel movements until his intestines emptied. Afterward, he shivered and curled up in bed for the next eight to twelve hours, afraid he was dying from a heart attack.

His doctor ordered a battery of tests, including a cardiac stress test and upper and lower GI scoping. Blood tests ruled out Lyme disease, and stool samples eliminated parasites as the cause of his symptoms. A twenty-four-hour urine collection tested for signs of inflammation, but the results were inconclusive.

Martin endured two frustrating years of testing. During that time, his baggy clothes hung on his body as he lost twenty pounds. He dreaded each doctor visit because he received the same news every time—the previous test was negative so he needed another one. Ultimately, all his results were negative, including a small intestine biopsy to rule out celiac disease.

On Martin's final visit, when the doctor didn't know what else to do, he suggested Martin try a gluten-free diet. Within two days Martin knew gluten *was the problem. He felt better than he had in two years. He was relieved to understand what caused his grueling symptoms after all this time and testing.*

If Martin ingests even a crumb of bread, his symptoms return with a vengeance. Martin has non-celiac gluten sensitivity. He must be vigilant to ensure his food is not cross-contaminated with anything that contains gluten.

———————————————

Do you think you might be gluten sensitive? Gluten-related disorders can cause more than two hundred different symptoms, most of which are not digestive. For example, my daughter suffered from headaches beginning in intermediate school. In college she experienced nosebleeds for the first time in her life. She only grew to five feet—a small stature. All of these symptoms derived from an intolerance to gluten, but none had anything to do with her gastrointestinal (GI) tract.

Gluten disorders can strike at any age. My friend Martin, whose story you just read, experienced heart-related symptoms associated with gluten. He'd consumed wheat his whole life without problems. However, later in life, intolerance to gluten caused him to suffer chest pains, similar to a heart attack.

Even if you tested negative for a gluten-related condition years ago, you could still develop it later in life. Figuring out whether you are sensitive to gluten or wheat is like putting together a challenging puzzle. Random pieces don't make sense and won't until the whole picture fits together.

Part of the difficulty is that conventional medicine has just begun to establish protocols for determining whether a person is gluten sensitive. In fact, only in 2010 was non-celiac gluten sensitivity recognized as a medical condition distinct from celiac disease.[1] Until recently, doctors lacked medical school education about this disorder.

To help you learn to solve your own gluten puzzle, chapter 1 defines each gluten-related condition (celiac disease, non-celiac gluten sensitivity, wheat sensitivity, and wheat allergy). Chapter 2 provides a checklist of symptoms for each condition so you can identify your symptoms. After utilizing the checklist, you will have a better understanding of your symptoms and how they might relate to these disorders. Whether you experience digestive or nondigestive symptoms that you don't understand, ruling out a gluten-related diagnosis will help you move one step closer to achieving your wellness.

My daughter complained of all sorts of nondigestive symptoms beginning in intermediate school but remained undiagnosed until her last year of college. Before 1980 it took an average of eleven years to be diagnosed. Currently, it still takes four.[2] Therefore, as healthcare consumers, wisdom dictates that we educate ourselves so we can improve our health. If you want to find out if you have a gluten-related disorder, you may need to ensure that your doctor orders the appropriate tests. I will outline the diagnostic criteria for each disorder in chapter 3.

If you find you have a gluten-related ailment, when you start the gluten-free diet you may feel better in a matter of days. Martin did. All of his symptoms resolved.

The second time my sister ate a gluten-free diet, she experienced success because the first time she tried it she didn't realize that gluten hides in numerous foods. For example, many salad dressings, condiments, and spices contain gluten. Trying to figure out how to become gluten-free may seem like a maze, but I will explain how in chapter 4.

The chapters open with true stories of individuals with a gluten-related disorder and their quest to solve their gluten puzzle. Varying in age, all of these people were poked, prodded, and administered stress tests, endoscopies, colonoscopies, and CAT scans. Some were diagnosed with other issues like Crohn's disease, irritable bowel syndrome, or colic. They suffered from low-birth weight, attention deficit disorder (ADD), and autoimmune diseases. Over time, all of them were finally diagnosed with a gluten-related condition. We will learn what symptoms these individuals experienced, why it took so long to obtain a diagnosis, and how they transitioned to being gluten-free. Their stories may help you identify your own symptoms.

Has your health declined or the health of a loved one spun out of control? What if intolerance to gluten is a factor and you don't know it? If gluten harms you, simply changing your diet might resolve your symptoms. Yes, it is difficult to give up bread and pasta, but well worth it to resolve the ensuing health issues. Chapter 5 will help you embrace the gluten-free lifestyle with joy. Think of the benefits of experiencing energy and clarity of mind, as well as eliminating mood swings, headaches, and digestive issues.

The gluten-free lifestyle is a new trend. Currently, hundreds of gluten-free products are available in grocery stores, and most items are clearly labeled. Chapter 6 helps you navigate stores, read labels, and plan menus. Fortunately nowadays, most restaurants carry gluten-free options on their menu. However, this was not the case a decade ago. We investigate the reason why gluten sensitivity skyrocketed.

Restaurants must be extremely careful that they do not cross-contaminate food made for someone with celiac disease or gluten sensitivity. Martin's intolerance to gluten is high. He has to keep a separate peanut butter jar and butter dish from the rest of the family so a knife that touches a slice of bread is not redipped into the jar. Cross-contamination from condiments at restaurants can easily occur. One of the gluten sensitive individuals I interviewed is a restaurant owner. In chapter 7, we discuss cross-contamination and eating out.

People with gluten-related ailments are a growing population. These individuals need to educate and equip themselves with the facts so they can take control of their health. That is why I wrote this book, so you can benefit from all I've learned personally and professionally about this puzzling disorder.

Have you complained about the same symptoms to different doctors with no answers? As consumers, we may need to guide our healthcare providers to rule out a gluten-related condition. Take this journey to determine whether your negative symptoms are caused by the inability to digest a protein called gluten. What do you have to lose but unwanted symptoms?

1

DEFINING GLUTEN-RELATED DISORDERS

Susan's Story

As a child I regularly blew my nose and snorted to clear the phlegm from my nasal passageways. My mother, annoyed by my repulsive habit, thought these symptoms might be an allergy, so she took me to an allergist. The doctor performed a painful skin prick test on my back.

I lay facedown on the examining table while the nurse stuck dozens of needles into my back. Itching ensued. I wanted to get up and run away but was forced to lie there and endure the allergic reactions on my back. The skin on my back erupted in a red, raised welt to the wheat allergen. The doctor diagnosed me with a wheat allergy.

Managing my allergy was challenging because gluten-free foods did not exist forty years ago. Most of our school lunches included a homemade yeast roll that was hard to resist. Sandwiches were a staple in that day and age. I continued to eat wheat and suffered from nasal congestion for years.

Fortunately, I grew out of the wheat allergy and my annoying snorting. As a young adult I did not experience unpleasant symptoms from eating wheat. However, at fifty, I suffered a health crisis where an abscessed tooth caused ten medical diagnoses and two surgeries in sixteen months. (See appendix 1 for the full story.)

After this illness, I had good days and bad. On the bad days, upon awak-

ening I couldn't think clearly and completely lacked motivation to accomplish anything. Cranky, irritable, and short-tempered, I knew my family also suffered from my symptoms.

It took a long time to figure out was wrong. Some days, exhaustion overwhelmed my body and fog incapacitated my brain. I thought I had chronic fatigue syndrome. I wanted to figure out what was wrong with me so I began a food journal. I documented what I ate twenty-four hours before each episode. I discovered that I consistently had eaten some form of wheat. Because I valued clarity of mind, a high energy level, and a well-balanced temperament, I chose not to eat wheat products.

I am wheat sensitive. I can eat products made with barley or rye with no adverse effects. Therefore, my diet is not as limited as someone with gluten sensitivity or celiac disease.

Gluten seems to be the boogeyman of the twenty-first century. Most of us know someone negatively affected by gluten. The diagnosis can range from a mild sensitivity to full-blown celiac. In this chapter we will define gluten, gluten-related disorders, and why these health issues have skyrocketed.

What exactly is gluten? Gluten is a protein found in the grains wheat, rye, and barley. The proteins in wheat are called glutenin and gliadin. The damage-causing protein in rye is secalin, and in barley it is hordein. These proteins are difficult for humans to digest. Even though the proteins are called different names, they all go by the umbrella term *gluten*. Therefore, even if your diet was wheat-free, it may not be gluten-free if you consume gluten from barley or rye.

Fifty years ago, gluten-related illnesses were rare. Today they are increasing at alarming rates, unexplained by genetic factors or an increased recognition of the disease. Therefore, some environmental factors must exist. One of the reasons for the rise in gluten-related conditions may be that the human body cannot proficiently digest the gluten in wheat because of the way it is hybridized today.

For centuries, people flourished by consuming bread. So why are we experiencing illness from this food today? The problem with modern wheat is that it is not processed the same as it was a hundred years ago. In 1970 Norman Borlaug received the Nobel Peace Prize in recognition of his contribution to world peace by increasing the global food supply through hybridization—crossbreeding of different varieties—of wheat.1

He crossbred various types of wheat to create a high-yield dwarf wheat. No longer do tall amber waves of grain grow in the Midwest. Instead, wheat is now only a couple of feet tall, drought-resistant, and prolific.2 Unfortunately, the gluten in the hybrid wheat changed so much that it became more difficult to digest, causing some individuals to become sensitive or intolerant to the gluten.3 In fact, older varieties of wheat, such as einkorn and emmer, may be better tolerated by those with a gluten-related condition than the current strains used in food production.

Whether a person has a known gluten-related disorder or not, the gluten molecule cannot be broken down completely by gastric enzymes. If a person's body does not recognize gluten as food, the immune system attacks the gluten and the body at the same time. The intestinal lining becomes damaged, resulting in holes in the intestinal wall (called leaky gut). Those holes allow food fragments to enter the bloodstream.4 Our bodies don't recognize these particles, so our immune system creates antibodies that cause food allergies (wheat allergy), gluten sensitivity, and autoimmune diseases (celiac disease) to develop.5

In turn, a person may become allergic to other types of food as well. It is not surprising that gluten sensitivity is often paired with an autoimmune condition, because the body accidentally harms its own cells as it attacks the broken-down food particles in the bloodstream.

Most Americans have no idea wheat has been bred to the point that the body attacks the gluten contained in it as a foreign substance. Hybridization is not the only enemy. What if the body also doesn't recognize genetically modified (GMO) food? Again, a person's immune system might attack the foreign substance and its own body simultaneously.

One type of genetically modified crop, Roundup Ready crops, are genetically engineered to be resistant to the carcinogen glyphosate—the primary ingredient in the herbicide Roundup. In the United States most of the nation's wheat, corn, soy, and oat crops are Roundup Ready crops.[6] Farmers who produce Roundup Ready crops are free to spray the herbicide on their fields throughout the growing season, as the plants are resistant. Therefore, a glyphosate residue may remain on the crop after harvest.

Can you imagine what this carcinogen (Roundup) may do to the beneficial bacteria in your gut or to your overall health? Your immune system may identify the GMO RoundUp Ready wheat as a foreign substance and accidentally injure your body while attacking the GMO wheat. In the past decade, the amount of RoundUp Ready crops has escalated. Therefore, I believe the rise in gluten-related conditions comes from the hybridization of wheat, the GMO Roundup Ready wheat crops, or both.

Gluten-Related Disorders

Celiac disease (CD), non-celiac gluten sensitivity (NCGS), wheat sensitivity, and wheat allergy are the four types of gluten-related disorders. Once considered rare, now gluten-related disorders affect nearly 10 percent of the population. With over seven billion people in the world, as many as 700 million could be affected by one of these conditions and not even know it. In some people, symptoms do not manifest until later in life—like Martin, whose story we read in the introduction.

Celiac Disease
Although CD has been recognized for more than one hundred

years, the link between CD and wheat consumption was not identified until the 1940s. A Dutch pediatrician, Willem K. Dicke, discovered his CD patients' symptoms improved during the bread shortages of World War II. Conversely, his patients relapsed when bread became readily available again. The gluten proteins in the wheat bread exacerbated his patients' symptoms.

Three conditions must exist for CD to develop:

1. Genetic predisposition
2. Environmental trigger
3. Consumption of gluten

A genetic test can be performed to determine if you carry the CD gene human leukocyte antigen HLA-DQ2 or HLA-DQ8. Thirty percent of the population carries the gene, but only 3 percent of individuals develop CD.[7] Studies demonstrated that first-degree relatives (sibling, parent, or child) of people with CD are at an increased risk of acquiring the disease.

The second factor necessary for CD to develop is a trigger. Celiac disease usually develops after some environmental factor such as illness, injury, pregnancy, surgery, or a major life event. Stressful significant life experiences include divorce, death of a loved one, emotional trauma, loss of a job, or even a move.

Worldwide, CD affects approximately 1 percent of the general population—that's 70 million people! Yet most have not been diagnosed. The prevalence of CD increased 400 percent in the past fifty to sixty years.[8] Is it a coincidence the hybridization of wheat occurred in the 1960s?

Celiac disease is the most severe form of a gluten-related disorder. It is an autoimmune disease where the body attacks the gluten molecule and mucosal lining of the small intestine simultaneously. The lining of the small intestine contains villi, hairlike projections that increase the surface of the intestinal lining, enabling a person to absorb nutrients from digested food effectively. The immune system's overactive, inflammatory response to gluten harms the villi, causing flattened, patchy sections in individuals with CD. Damaged villi no longer effectively absorb nutrients from food.

The gold standard for diagnosing CD is an endoscopy that obtains a small bowel biopsy of the villi. Unfortunately, this is not a perfect science, as it may be difficult to locate the patchy areas of damaged villi in the gastrointestinal tract. Therefore, an initial biopsy is accurate only 65 percent of the time.[9] Several biopsies may be necessary to confirm the presence of harmed villi.

Celiac disease is difficult to recognize because it causes a wide variety of symptoms. At this time, more CD patients experience nondigestive issues such as fatigue, brain fog, joint pain, rash, eczema, headache, anxiety, or depression than the classic malabsorption symptoms of diarrhea. These nondigestive symptoms make it more difficult for physicians to detect and diagnose CD.

Different autoimmune diseases such as type 1 diabetes and thyroid diseases like Hashimoto's and Graves' are associated with CD. In fact, the longer a person goes undiagnosed, the more likely the immune system will harm other areas of the body, causing another autoimmune disorder to occur. About 6 percent of people with type 1 diabetes have CD. Similar to CD, type 1 diabetes occurs when a person's immune system harms their pancreas, causing an inability to produce insulin. An overactive immune system could also damage the thyroid of someone with CD.

Treatment of CD includes a strict gluten-free diet. However, if a person with CD eats a gluten-free diet before testing, the results will most likely be false-negative because when you stop consuming gluten, your body stops making antibodies against it (see chapter 3). Therefore, ask your doctor to test you before you stop eating foods containing gluten. The good news is that once a person with CD eliminates gluten from their diet, their small intestine heals (most of the time). Our bodies are programmed to heal themselves—like the natural healing of a cut or sprained ankle. The small intestine can heal completely if the disease is caught early and the person stops eating gluten.

A CD diagnosis may seem devastating; however, it is not as serious or life-threatening as surgery or a malignancy. Instead the disease is treated through diet modification. While such a lifestyle change is a significant adjustment, on the bright side, someone with CD needs no therapeutic treatments or medications to recover. Read chapter 5 to learn how to embrace the gluten-free lifestyle positively.

Gluten Sensitivity

Non-celiac gluten sensitivity (NCGS) is the term currently used to describe individuals who react to gluten without meeting the diagnostic criteria for CD or an allergy to wheat. NCGS became a clinical condition distinct from celiac disease in 2010.[10] Therefore, this condition is a brand-new diagnosis countless people have not heard about and do not understand. An estimated 3–6 percent of the human population—up to 420 million people worldwide—are affected. Currently, no specific test to diagnose NCGS exists, but researchers are working to develop one.

Needless to say, NCGS is challenging to diagnose. Many individuals attempt to self-diagnose by eliminating gluten from their diet. If their symptoms subside, they were suffering from CD, NCGS, wheat sensitivity, or a wheat allergy. However, if symptoms continue, their specific problem is not caused by gluten, or they may not have completely eliminated gluten from their diet because it is hidden in so many common foods.

The good thing about NCGS is that the small intestine is not damaged as it is with CD. Gluten sensitivity occurs in varying degrees, from mild to highly sensitive. Martin is an example of a person who is highly gluten sensitive. Someone with a mild sensitivity may be able to ingest small amounts of gluten and not react negatively.

If you experience symptoms of a gluten-related illness, ask your physician to test you. Again, make sure you are tested before giving up gluten. Remember, blood test results are invalid if you are not consuming gluten at the time of the blood draw.

Wheat Sensitivity

A spectrum of gluten-related disorders exists. On one end we find celiac disease and on the opposite end a wheat allergy (see next section). Part of the gray area between CD and wheat allergy is wheat sensitivity. For wheat sensitivity, the person reacts to wheat, but the reaction is not an autoimmune response (CD) or an allergic reaction (wheat allergy).

With wheat sensitivity, gluten from barley or rye is not the problem. Only the gluten from wheat is the culprit. I am wheat sensitive. The day after I eat bread I feel tired and foggy brained. However, I can consume barley (similar to rice), beer, and malt vinegar made from barley, without any problems. Therefore, I do not have as restricted a diet as Martin. Maybe I became sensitive to wheat because I was allergic to wheat as a child but continued to eat it.

A person may think they are NCGS when in fact the sensitivity could be solely due to wheat. The gluten protein in modern, hybridized wheat is larger and more difficult to digest. Chapter 3 outlines the steps to differentiate between gluten sensitivity and wheat sensitivity.

Wheat Allergy

The last category of a gluten-related disorder is a wheat allergy. Wheat is one of the most common food allergens in the US. An allergy to wheat is more common in children and can affect up to 1 percent of the population. Resolution of the allergy occurs in 65 percent of children by the age of twelve.[11]

A wheat allergy occurs when someone experiences an allergic reaction to food containing wheat. This is not an allergy to gluten. The reaction arises as an immune response when the body's defense system overreacts. An allergic reaction occurs within minutes to a few hours. Symptoms may range from mild to severe and could result in anaphylactic shock—a life-threatening condition.

An allergy to wheat is different from CD, NCGS, and wheat sensitivity. The following diagram displays the spectrum of gluten-related disorders. In the next chapter, we will discuss the diagnostic tests used to determine each condition.

Celiac Disease-Gluten Sensitivity—Wheat Sensitivity—Wheat Allergy

Summary

You should now have a clear understanding of each of the four gluten-related disorders—celiac disease, non-celiac gluten sensitivity, wheat sensitivity, and wheat allergy. Next we will review the symptoms for each of these conditions. Determining what caused your symptoms and which diagnosis you may have is the puzzle you need to solve. Researchers and doctors have not yet fully unscrambled the puzzle, but they are working on it.

SYMPTOMS OF GLUTEN-RELATED DISORDERS

Tonya's Story

At birth Tonya weighed a mere five pounds. Despite being breastfed in the first month, she did not gain weight. So the doctor recommended Tonya's mother use formula.

After switching, Tonya cried constantly and suffered from diarrhea. Her parents tried every baby formula on the market, hoping to resolve her digestive issues. She tolerated none, and all her family members were baptized with Tonya's pale, runny stools.

Running out of options, Tonya's mother took her back to the pediatrician, who diagnosed colic (severe abdominal pain caused by gas). Around Tonya's first birthday, her mother, disillusioned with formula, gave her daughter watered-down juice, which helped a little.

As she grew, no matter what her mother served, Tonya ate very little. Her parents encouraged her, "Take one more bite." The times she tried, it often backfired, and she vomited her food immediately. Tonya's stomach consistently ached after meals. Diarrhea followed.

At age seven Tonya weighed a dismal thirty-seven pounds. As a child, her low weight never registered on the growth scale. The pattern of regurgitation, abdominal pain, and diarrhea carried on throughout her childhood until *puberty, when she finally began to grow. Surprisingly her symptoms went away, and she became athletic.*

When she entered college, Tonya seemed in good health and even ventured out into the college lifestyle. Cocktails and wine were tolerable, but beer brought on her old illness. Otherwise she rarely had digestive issues. She graduated with a bachelor's degree in nursing.

At age twenty-five, Tonya began to notice that various foods and drinks caused nausea and severe abdominal pain. Tonya didn't understand why she suffered from these symptoms, because they had basically gone away since puberty, so she saw her family doctor. He determined she was anemic and malnourished, and he referred her to a gastroenterologist, who prescribed gastroesophageal reflux medication (antacids) and vitamins. However, Tonya continued to experience intermittent bouts of diarrhea and constipation.

About that time, Tonya's mother was hospitalized for a twenty-seven-pound weight loss during a two-week episode of severe vomiting, diarrhea, and abdominal pain—similar symptoms to what Tonya experienced earlier in her life. Upon hospital admission, Tonya's mother learned she suffered from malnutrition and pernicious anemia (a deficiency in red blood cells from a lack of vitamin B_{12}). As the physician started Tonya's mother's diagnostic workup, he suspected cancer, but upon obtaining biopsies of her small intestine, cancer was ruled out. Instead, she tested positive for celiac disease.

Around age twenty-seven Tonya experienced some normalcy in life. She was married and working full time as an intensive care unit nurse. She consistently ran three miles several times a week and played on a recreational volleyball league.

Unexpectedly, Tonya began to vomit daily after every meal for a month. She had to have a bathroom or trashcan close by all the time. After an onset of piercing abdominal pain, Tonya was rushed to the emergency room and then admitted to the hospital.

She suffered from autoimmune pancreatitis. Tonya's immune system attacked her pancreas, causing nausea, vomiting, and excruciating abdominal pain. In addition, the doctor diagnosed her with Hashimoto's thyroid disease. She needed surgery to remove her gallbladder too.

Tonya remained hospitalized for a grueling six months while she received total parenteral nutrition (TPN)—a method of infusing a nutritional substance directly into her veins around the clock. She was not allowed food or drink.

During this time she experienced every possible emotion—fear, anger, self-pity, depression, and hopelessness. Fortunately, she had a strong support system with her husband, parents, and siblings. They didn't waver from their love, encouragement, patience, and faith. When Tonya's faith was tested most, her friends and family always found a way to rejuvenate it. Ultimately, she realized how fortunate she truly was to have all of them despite her medical predicament.

While hospitalized, she asked her doctor to test her for celiac disease because of her mother's recent diagnosis. At that time blood tests for celiac disease did not exist; it was only diagnosed through a biopsy of the jejunal portion of the small intestine. Her doctor could not perform an endoscopy because her diagnosis of pancreatitis precluded it. Also, the TPN did not contain gluten, so the biopsy might not have been accurate.

A week before discharge, Tonya transitioned to a clear-liquid diet. After her release she tried a gluten-free diet, but she still experienced occasional digestive issues. She was never able to return to volleyball or running, but she began working again a month later. Abdominal pain and diarrhea persisted when she consumed carbohydrates and raw vegetables. She thought her intermittent symptoms might be due to her gallbladder removal.

Finally, at twenty-nine and still in search of answers to her lifelong struggles, Tonya saw her gastroenterologist, who performed an endoscopy and biopsied her small intestine. The result: stage 4 celiac disease like her mother. Stage 4, the most advanced phase of the disease, occurs when the villi are completely flattened. Tonya felt relief in finally being diagnosed but was still far from a normal life. Her physician encouraged her to eat a strict gluten-free diet. Unfortunately, symptoms of abdominal pain, nausea, bloating, and diarrhea persisted.

Three years later, her gastroenterologist performed an upper endoscopy, which confirmed that her gastrointestinal (GI) tract never healed despite her gluten-free diet. Therefore, her diagnosis progressed to refractory celiac disease—a complex autoimmune disorder that is unresponsive to twelve months of treatment on a strict gluten-free diet. Sadly, Tonya's flattened villi *cannot absorb nutrients, and she continues to suffer from malabsorption and GI symptoms.*

As a result of the autoimmune thyroid disease—Hashimoto's—she had a total thyroidectomy at age thirty-six. Occasionally, she experiences an autoimmune pancreatitis flare-up. Her most recent diagnosis is multiple sclerosis, another autoimmune disease. When celiac disease is untreated or not diagnosed early, it can lead to severe health problems.

————————————

At this point, you understand why figuring out if you have a gluten-related disorder is like solving a puzzle. Honestly, I did not fully appreciate my wheat sensitivity diagnosis until I completed my scientific research for this book. Nonetheless, I knew I suffered from different symptoms than my sister, as she is highly non-celiac gluten sensitive (NCGS). Her story is presented in chapter 5.

Tonya suffered for twenty-nine years before her diagnosis, even though she exhibited symptoms from birth. Not long ago CD was rarely diagnosed. In fact, only recently has the medical establishment discovered the full spectrum of gluten-related disorders.

The medical community recognized they were not keeping up. To remedy this, a task force of sixteen physicians from seven countries met in Oslo, Norway. Their purpose was to define each gluten-related disorder. They published their conclusions in 2013. *Solving the Gluten Puzzle* uses the most current definitions from the task force.

The Oslo recommendations created the term *gluten-related disorders* to describe the different medical conditions related to the ingestion of gluten. This includes celiac disease, non-celiac gluten sensitivity, and other related illnesses.

In addition to the Oslo task force, the US Preventative Services Task Force commissioned a report to determine recommendations for celiac disease screening in persons three years or older. The

Journal of the American Medical Association published the report in 2017. It concluded that little or no evidence existed to screen for CD in asymptomatic individuals. Since gluten-related conditions can develop at any point in a person's life, it didn't make sense to test someone until they exhibited symptoms, or if they had a first-degree relative (parent, sibling, or child) with CD.

Unless physicians read pertinent and updated information or attend conferences that address gluten-related disorders, they may be unaware of the new terminology or myriad of symptoms now recognized from gluten-related disorders. You can guide your physician by asking to be tested for a gluten-related condition if you suspect you have one (see the gluten quiz at SusanUNeal.com/GlutenQuiz).

Celiac Disease Definitions and Symptoms

The following list of CD definitions developed from the Oslo medical task force. The task force performed a literature review of scientific studies conducted from 1900–2011. Their recommended definitions created a foundation for the treatment of patients with CD.

Asymptomatic celiac disease occurs when an individual has CD but does not experience symptoms. Sometimes these individuals do not recognize they felt minor symptoms—such as fatigue, acid reflux, abdominal bloating, and flatulence—until they eat a gluten-free diet. Diagnosing asymptomatic CD primarily occurs when individuals obtain testing due to a relative's recent diagnosis. A family member's CD diagnosis means relatives are at a higher risk of developing the disease. Even without symptoms, someone with asymptomatic CD is at risk for long-term complications.

Celiac disease has a genetic component, and when you have a first-degree relative with the disease, your chances of developing CD are 8–15 percent.[1] The company 23andMe (https://blog.23andme.com/health-traits/new-23andme-report-celiac-disease/) has a celiac disease genetic test. The test identifies the two genes—human leukocyte antigen HLA-DQ2 and HLA-DQ8—that account for 95 percent of CD cases. Carrying one of these genes doesn't mean you will develop CD. Thirty percent of the population has the gene, while only 3 percent develop the disease. If you don't carry a CD gene, it is highly unlikely you will develop CD.

Potential CD refers to individuals who tested positive for the gene or have a first-degree relative diagnosed with CD. It also includes patients who had a negative small intestine biopsy but positive blood test results. Since the blood test reveals antibodies against gluten, these individuals could develop the disease later if they continue to consume gluten.

Classic CD occurs when an individual demonstrates signs of malabsorption. With malabsorption, significant damage to the small intestine occurred to the point where the body cannot effectively absorb the nutrients in food. Classic symptoms include diarrhea, weight loss, malnutrition, abdominal pain, and anemia. Also, the person may have large, foul-smelling stools that contain fat, with a pale, oily appearance. This is due to the failure to properly digest and absorb food. In children, this could be misdiagnosed as failure to thrive. Children may experience abdominal distention, poor appetite, lethargy, and moodiness.

In the past, medical training programs taught physicians to identify CD based upon classic symptoms. Even though Tonya exhibited classic symptoms of CD, she was misdiagnosed.

In *nonclassic CD* the person does not suffer from malabsorption of nutrients. Instead, the symptoms are not gastrointestinal but range across a broad spectrum of indications. It is no wonder that many physicians do not attribute a nongastrointestinal complaint as a sign of CD, because these symptoms are not associated with classic CD. The following list includes many of the CD symptoms for both classic and nonclassic, separated into GI and nongastrointestinal categories.

Celiac Disease Gastrointestinal Symptoms

Put a check by the following symptoms you experience:

_____ Nausea

_____ Vomiting

_____ Burping

_____ Acid reflux or gastroesophageal reflux disease (GERD)

_____ Heartburn

_____ Stomach rumbling

_____ Gas and flatulence

_____ Bloating

_____ Abdominal distension

_____ Abdominal pain

_____ Constipation

_____ Diarrhea

_____ Mushy stools

_____ Smelly stools

_____ Floating stools

_____ Pale, oily stools

_____ Bulky or loose stools

_____ Irritable bowel syndrome

_____ Voracious appetite

_____ Weight gain

_____ Stomach problems (atrophic gastritis)

_____ Microscopic colitis

_____ Lymphocytic colitis

_____ Digestive cancer (intestinal lymphoma)

_____ Gastrointestinal cancer

Celiac Disease Nongastrointestinal Symptoms

Put a check by the following unhealthy symptoms you experience:

_____ Acne

_____ Rash

_____ Eczema

_____ Rosacea

_____ Psoriasis

_____ Dermatitis herpetiformis (itchy skin rash)

_____ Canker sores (mouth sores)

_____ Cracking of the corner of the mouth

_____ Bruising

_____ Hair loss

_____ Nosebleeds

_____ Dry eyes

_____ Discolored teeth

_____ Dental enamel defects

_____ Lactose intolerance

_____ Poor appetite

_____ Weight loss

_____ Malnutrition

_____ Iron deficient anemia

_____ Vitamin and/or mineral deficiency (low folic acid, B_{12}, etc.)

_____ Delayed growth

_____ Delayed puberty

_____ Failure to thrive

_____ Short stature

_____ Muscle wasting

_____ Muscle cramping

_____ Bone or muscle pain

_____ Aching, painful joints (hands, shoulders, elbows, wrists, knees, spine, hips)

_____ Arthritis

_____ Rheumatoid arthritis

_____ Weakness

_____ Generalized loss of strength

_____ Clumsiness

_____ Decline in hand coordination

_____ Poor balance and coordination

_____ Peripheral ataxia (trouble moving parts of the body, including hands, feet, arms, and legs)

_____ Peripheral neuropathy (weakness, tingling, numbness, and pain in the hands and feet)

_____ Fractures (weak bones)

_____ Osteopenia

_____ Osteoporosis

_____ Anxiety

_____ Panic attacks

_____ Irritability

_____ Moodiness

_____ Depression

_____ Mood disorders

_____ Behavioral issues

_____ Attention deficit disorder (ADD)

_____ Attention deficit hyperactivity disorder (ADHD)

_____ Autistic type behavior

_____ Lack of motivation

_____ Fatigue/tiredness

_____ Chronic fatigue syndrome

_____ Swelling (edema)

_____ Inflammation

_____ Fibromyalgia

_____ Autoimmune disorder

_____ Autoimmune hepatitis

_____ Sjogren's syndrome

_____ Hashimoto's disease

_____ Graves' disease

_____ Lupus erythematosus

_____ Gluten ataxia (autoimmune disorder that attacks the brain)

_____ Infertility

_____ Low sperm count

_____ Low testosterone

_____ Abnormal menstrual cycle

_____ Absence of menstruation

_____ Recurrent fetal loss (miscarriage)

_____ Intrauterine growth retardation (slow growth of a fetus)

_____ Night vision problems

_____ Headache

_____ Migraine

_____ Foggy brain

_____ Inability to concentrate and focus
_____ Neurological symptoms
_____ Cognitive and memory problems
_____ Seizures
_____ White spots on the brain
_____ Loss of grey matter in the brain
_____ Shrinking of the brain's cerebellum
_____ Shrunken spleen
_____ Kidney disease
_____ Thyroid disease
_____ Abnormal liver function test (elevated liver enzymes)
_____ Low blood sugar (hypoglycemia)
_____ Lung disorders (fibrosis and sarcoidosis)
_____ Heart-related conditions (cardiomyopathy and myocarditis)
_____ Liver and biliary tract disorders (transaminitis, fatty liver, primary sclerosing cholangitis)

How many puzzle pieces did you identify in this list? If you experience several of these symptoms, you should let your physician know. However, many of these symptoms can be caused by different health problems other than celiac disease. Your physician can help you figure that out.

Two celiac websites provide questionnaires you can complete to determine your likelihood of having CD. After you complete the assessment, the website emails you the results. The celiac.org website provides a letter for you to give to your physician with the symptoms that indicate you are at an increased risk for CD. Here are the links:

Celiac.org/about-celiac-disease/symptoms-assessment-tool/
Beyondceliac.org/celiac-disease/symptoms-checklist/

After reviewing the CD symptom list, you can understand the difficulty in diagnosing it. Celiac disease affects an astonishing number of bodily systems. A gastroenterologist understands CD and recognizes the two-hundred-plus symptoms associated with it.

However, a primary care physician may not attribute some of these symptoms to CD, so you may need to seek out a specialist.

Currently, it is estimated that one in a hundred Americans have CD, but less than 20 percent are diagnosed.[2] Therefore, approximately 80 percent of CD individuals do not know they have the disease. The Celiac Disease Foundation website states, "A lack of training in medical schools and primary care residency programs, contribute to the poor diagnosis rate in the United States."[3] The following CD symptoms are explained in detail to provide further understanding.

Weight Gain

Forty percent of Americans suffer from obesity. Could this have anything to do with CD? Some individuals with CD have voracious appetites because they are not absorbing the nutrients in food. They lack essential vitamins, minerals, and micronutrients, so their body craves more food to try to gain the nourishment they require. Unfortunately, the person still isn't able to absorb the deficient nutrients, but they consumed all the calories, which caused excessive weight gain.

Infertility

What does CD have to do with infertility? CD causes a low sperm count and low levels of the male hormone testosterone. Several studies found a higher incidence of CD in women with unexplained infertility and pregnancy issues, including repeated miscarriages and low birth weights. Therefore, if a couple is having difficulty getting pregnant, they should ask their physician to test them for CD.

Brain and Nervous System Disorders

Celiac disease can affect the brain by causing shrinking of the cerebellum, loss of gray matter, white spots on the brain, and memory and cognition problems. Vitamin and mineral deficiencies for an extended period, due to the body's inability to absorb food, could contribute to these abnormalities. Alternatively, the body's overactive immune system may attack the brain and nervous system like it does the small intestine.

Irritable Bowel Syndrome

A common misdiagnosis for CD is irritable bowel syndrome. Both have similar symptoms that include gas, bloating, abdominal pain, and diarrhea. A single diagnostic test to determine IBS or gluten sensitivity does not exist. Therefore, a doctor may think you have irritable bowel syndrome because this disorder upsets the way your bowels function, but it does not cause long-term damage to your intestinal tract like CD.

Bones

If a person with CD is not absorbing essential nutrients like calcium and vitamin D, bone density is affected. Therefore, the compactness of the bones may be compromised, causing recurrent fractures, osteopenia (low bone mineral density), and osteoporosis. Once a person stops eating gluten, and the small intestine heals, most often he or she can absorb nutrients properly again, particularly if caught at an earlier stage.

Autoimmune Disorders

An autoimmune disease occurs when the body's immune system overreacts and harms the body, causing damage and inflammation. People with CD tend to develop other autoimmune conditions such as lupus, Hashimoto's, and Graves' thyroid diseases; Sjogren's syndrome; and rheumatoid arthritis. Tonya developed Hashimoto's disease in her midtwenties before being diagnosed with CD. If you have an autoimmune disease, you should be tested for CD. If you have

CD, the longer you eat gluten, the more likely you are to develop another autoimmune disorder.

The Celiac Disease Foundation website displayed a chart: "Early Diagnosis Lowers Chance for Developing Another Condition." The chart lists the age of diagnosis along with the statistical chance of developing another autoimmune condition (Celiac.org/about-celiac-disease/what-is-celiac-disease/). Tonya, who was diagnosed after age twenty, had a 34 percent chance of getting another autoimmune disease.

Dermatitis Herpetiformis

Dermatitis herpetiformis is an itchy, blistery skin rash that affects some individuals who have CD. The outbreak looks similar to herpes simplex (cold sore), but is not the same. It usually appears on the elbows, knees, buttocks, scalp, and back of the neck, but it can also appear on other parts of the body. Only people with CD have this skin condition. To diagnose dermatitis herpetiformis, a doctor takes a biopsy of the skin near the lesion to determine if it contains the IgA antibody (we will discuss testing in the next chapter). A gluten-free diet cures this skin condition.

Bowel Movements

Let's discuss an uncomfortable topic—bowel movements (BM). Variation in bowel movements ranges from three times a week to three times a day. However, it is best to expel a BM every day. During a lifetime, the frequency and pattern of BMs change. Stools are directly affected by how much fiber and water you consume. Low fiber and water intake contribute to constipation.

Normal stools can range in appearance from looking like sausage-shaped Milk Duds to a banana. Ideally your stool should pass easily and not be watery. Search the Internet for the Bristol Stool Chart to learn more. What you eat affects the appearance of your BM. Let your physician know if you suffer from symptoms listed under *classic CD* (diarrhea; abdominal pain and distension; foul-smelling, bulky stools containing fat, or which are pale and oily in appearance).

Test before Eating a Gluten-Free Diet

If you experience CD symptoms, get tested before trying a gluten-free diet. If you have not eaten gluten for over a month, hold off on testing until you consume gluten daily for several weeks. Otherwise, your test results may be false-negative, reflecting the absence of gluten in your diet and antibodies in your blood.

Early Diagnosis

When someone is diagnosed with CD early in the disease process and chooses to stop consuming gluten, most of the severe complications can be prevented. Talk to your doctor about your symptoms. An individual with CD can live a symptom-free life, even as long as someone who does not have the disease. The treatment is a strict gluten-free diet, and through this new lifestyle the symptoms usually resolve.

This was not the case for Tonya. It took so long for her to be diagnosed (age twenty-nine) that her small intestine never healed. Consequently, she developed refractory celiac disease, which is unresponsive to a gluten-free diet, and multiple sclerosis, another autoimmune disease. She continues to suffer from GI symptoms and malabsorption.

Refractory Celiac Disease

About 1–2 percent of those diagnosed with CD have an unresponsive form of the disease.[4] Refractory CD is a complex autoimmune disorder that does not respond to twelve months of treatment on a strict gluten-free diet. The villi in the small intestine do not heal. Generally, this form of CD occurs in adults over fifty, and the symptoms are usually more severe.

Scientists do not understand why refractory celiac disease develops. However, it may result from having CD and consuming gluten for numerous years before diagnosis, or the person may carry both human leukocyte antigen genes instead of only one. More research needs to occur to figure this out and help patients with this condition.

Non-Celiac Gluten Sensitivity Definition and Symptoms

Non-celiac gluten sensitivity is a condition where the ingestion of gluten leads to symptoms similar to celiac disease despite the absence of CD. Fortunately, the immune response in NCGS does not damage the villi in the small intestine. It is difficult to diagnose because blood tests for gluten antibodies are negative in over 80 percent of NCGS individuals.[5]

The most common NCGS symptoms based upon a review of 6,000 patients are: [6]

- Abdominal pain (70 percent suffered with this symptom)
- Eczema and/or rash (40 percent)
- Migraine headache (35 percent)
- Foggy mind (34 percent)
- Chronic fatigue (33 percent)
- Diarrhea (33 percent)
- Depression (22 percent)
- Anemia (20 percent)
- Tingling of fingertips (20 percent)
- Joint pain (11 percent)

The symptoms of NCGS are listed below. They are separated into gastrointestinal and nongastrointestinal symptoms.

. . .

Non-Celiac Gluten Sensitivity Gastrointestinal Symptoms

Put a check by the following unhealthy symptoms you experience:

_____ Nausea

_____ Vomiting

_____ Burping

_____ Acid reflux or gastroesophageal reflux disease (GERD)

_____ Heartburn

_____ Stomach rumbling

_____ Gas and flatulence

_____ Bloating

_____ Abdominal distension

_____ Abdominal pain

_____ Constipation

_____ Diarrhea

_____ Oily stools

_____ Smelly stools

_____ Floating stools

_____ Irritable bowel syndrome

Non-Celiac Gluten Sensitivity Nongastrointestinal Symptoms

Put a check by the following unhealthy symptoms you experience:

_____ Acne

_____ Rash

_____ Eczema

_____ Rosacea

_____ Psoriasis

_____ Canker sores (mouth sores)

_____ Bruising

_____ Hair loss

_____ Nosebleeds

_____ Dental enamel defects

_____ Lactose intolerance

_____ Weight loss

_____ Iron deficient anemia

_____ Vitamin and/or mineral deficiency

_____ Weight gain

_____ Muscle cramping

_____ Osteoporosis

_____ Bone pain

_____ Aching, painful joints

_____ Weakness

_____ Clumsiness

_____ Muscle control problems

_____ Poor balance and coordination

_____ Peripheral neuropathy (weakness, tingling, numbness, and pain in the hands and feet)

_____ Anxiety

_____ Irritability

_____ Moodiness

_____ Depression

_____ Mood disorders

_____ Attention deficit disorder (ADD)

_____ Attention deficit hyperactivity disorder (ADHD)

_____ Lack of motivation

_____ Fatigue/tiredness

_____ Swelling (Edema)

_____ Inflammation

_____ Autoimmune disorder

_____ Sjogren's syndrome

_____ Hashimoto's disease

_____ Lupus erythematosus

_____ Infertility

_____ Abnormal menstrual cycle

_____ Night vision problems

_____ Headache

_____ Migraine

_____ Foggy brain

_____ Inability to concentrate and focus

_____ Neurological symptoms

_____ Seizures
_____ Abnormal liver function test
_____ Low blood sugar (hypoglycemia)

The NCGS list of symptoms is not as long as it is for CD. However, these symptoms can turn a person's life upside down. I know it did for my sister; she was hospitalized for low potassium because of chronic diarrhea. This essential electrolyte dropped life threateningly low. As a result, for the rest of her life she has to take blood pressure medication to prevent her body from getting the "shakes." Has your life been affected by NCGS symptoms? If so, please let your physician know so he can test you.

The symptoms you experience with NCGS may be completely different from someone else. Martin's symptoms resembled a heart attack. My sister experienced GI symptoms. I suffered from brain fog and exhaustion.

The level of sensitivity is different for each person with NCGS. Martin is highly sensitive. He can't have any exposure to gluten without severe health consequences. Conversely, I know other NCGS individuals who can handle ingesting a little gluten from time to time with minor unpleasant effects.

A typical nerve-related symptom of CD and NCGS is peripheral neuropathy. This is a dysfunction of a nerve in an extremity (hand, foot, leg, or arm). The manifestation begins gradually and occurs infrequently. It is difficult to explain to a physician, or family member, that occasionally your hand goes numb or is hard to lift. These on-again, off-again symptoms can make you wonder if you're crazy. No, you are not. These symptoms are real, and loved ones and physicians should listen to you!

The nature of CD and NCGS randomly occurs, so you can't predict what will be affected. Are you clumsy? My daughter was. As a child she seemed to frequently fall off her chair at the dinner table, as an adolescent she often tripped, and as a teenager she repeatedly dropped food on her shirt.

Celiac disease and non-celiac gluten sensitivity can cause a decline in hand coordination (spilled food on your shirt), difficulty with balancing/walking (tripping), and a generalized loss of strength. If CD or NCGS is causing you similar nerve-related symptoms, the sooner you switch to a gluten-free diet the better. Removing gluten can stabilize or eliminate these symptoms. However, the longer you go undiagnosed and continue to consume gluten, the more difficult it becomes for your body to heal.

The incidence of NCGS is higher than CD. It is estimated that gluten sensitivity affects between 3–6 percent of the human population—up to 420 million people worldwide. Do you think you may have NCGS?

Wheat Sensitivity Symptoms

Individuals who are sensitive to wheat may not be sensitive to gluten. They may be able to ingest foods that contain gluten when the source comes from barley or rye. A person with wheat sensitivity, like me, does not have as limited of a diet as someone with CD or NCGS.

The symptoms of wheat sensitivity are similar to the list of NCGS symptoms. If you have not done so already, please complete the NCGS checklist. If you experience NCGS symptoms, you may have a wheat sensitivity instead of a gluten sensitivity. We will discuss how to distinguish between the two in chapter 3.

Wheat Allergy Symptoms

Common allergic symptoms include sneezing, nasal congestion, coughing, throat tightness, and asthma. As a child, I experienced persistent nasal congestion. Do you experience any of the following symptoms after you eat wheat products?

. . .

Put a check by the following unhealthy symptoms you experience:

_____ Sneezing

_____ Coughing

_____ Nasal congestion

_____ Metallic taste in the mouth

_____ Itching, swelling, or irritation of the lips, tongue, throat, or other body parts

_____ Throat tightness

_____ Trouble swallowing

_____ Difficulty breathing

_____ Dizziness

_____ Fainting

_____ Pale skin color

_____ Rash

_____ Hives

_____ Nausea

_____ Indigestion

_____ Abdominal cramps

_____ Vomiting

_____ Diarrhea

_____ Muscle spasms

_____ Agitated feeling

_____ Drop in blood pressure

_____ Rapid heartbeat

_____ Chest pain or tightness

Exposure to an allergen can sometimes be life-threatening. For example, peanut allergies became more prevalent in the past two decades. All food brought into public school classrooms requires labeling of the ingredients because some children could react if they were in the same room with foods containing peanuts. Allergies can cause a person to go into anaphylaxis. If someone goes into anaphylaxis (anaphylactic shock) they need treatment immediately (call 911).

· · ·

Signs of Anaphylactic Shock

Usually, the response begins with a tingling or itching in the mouth and could include swelling of the lips, throat, or tongue. Other symptoms include:

_____ Dizziness or fainting

_____ Rapid heartbeat

_____ Swelling of the throat

_____ Severe difficulty breathing

_____ Pale blue skin color

_____ Chest pain

If these symptoms occur, call 911, as it could be a life-threatening emergency.

Symptom Tolerance

Sometimes we experience symptoms for so long we get used to them and think they are normal—like belching or reflux. However, the symptoms listed in this chapter are not normal. For example, I experienced iron-deficiency anemia all my life. I donated blood only once. My hemoglobin level was always too low to meet the minimum standard for donors. Since college I've taken daily iron supplements. I never considered my anemia as abnormal. My wheat allergy and sensitivity may have affected my ability to absorb this essential mineral.

Journal

Many of us have tolerated our symptoms for so long that we don't know what normal feels like anymore. Therefore, if you suffer from some of the symptoms listed in this chapter, I recommend keeping a food journal and tracking your corresponding symptoms. My food diary helped me understand that wheat products caused my fatigue and brain fog. I published *Healthy Living Journal* to help people identify food culprits. It can help you too.

In this journal you will spend a few minutes daily recording your food choices and how your body responds. With time you will see how different foods affect you physically, mentally, and emotionally. As you record and reflect in this journal, you will move one step closer to solving your gluten health puzzle.

Next time you see your doctor, take the journal with you. It will help you easily identify your symptoms. Many times you are under pressure to answer questions quickly during a medical appointment. The journal entries you recorded will provides those answers and eliminate the stress.

Summary

This chapter helped you gain knowledge regarding the signs and symptoms of CD, NCGS, wheat sensitivity, and a wheat allergy. Through identifying your symptoms, you know whether it's possible that you have one of these conditions. Next, we will learn the diagnostic tests used to diagnose each gluten-related disorder.

DIAGNOSTIC TESTS TO SOLVE THE GLUTEN PUZZLE

Amber's Story

During Amber's first year of college, she gained more than the "freshman ten." Ugh, she added twenty pounds. In her sophomore year she experienced stomach issues. Sometimes after a meal she felt pain in her gut, and had to run to the bathroom.

As these episodes continued, she usually thought that hot sauce or fried food upset her stomach, or she'd caught a stomach virus. She always found an excuse for her abdominal pain and diarrhea. As her symptoms persisted, she lost weight. During the Christmas holidays her family noticed she'd lost her "freshman twenty." She didn't tell anyone about her chronic diarrhea. Instead, she ignored it.

Her symptoms worsened during the second semester. Sometimes merely sipping on a soda caused her to go to the bathroom before eating her meal. Once she began eating, after several bites she experienced diarrhea again. Amber had difficulty consuming anything because of relentless interruptions from diarrhea.

As the semester continued, she regularly endured three or four bouts of diarrhea before finishing a meal. Her weight continued to drop.

At this point it was hard for Amber to function due to her chronic abdominal pain and diarrhea during meals. Between her classes, part-time job, and

GI symptoms, exhaustion enveloped her. At the end of her sophomore year, she packed and moved home to stay. She was too sick to continue attending college. She felt utter defeat and was unsure about her future.

When she returned home, her parents were extremely concerned for her well-being. She was thin as a rail, ghostly white, and slept all the time. They took her to a gastroenterologist.

Amber explained her symptoms to the doctor. He ordered the following blood tests and obtained these results:

- *Complete blood count (CBC)—normal except bilirubin was high*
- *Comprehensive metabolic panel—normal*
- *Vitamin B$_{12}$—low range of normal*
- *Tissue transglutaminase antibody (tTG-IgA)—negative*
- *Gliadin antibody (deamidated) (IgA and IgG)—negative*
- *C-reactive protein—normal*
- *H-pylori antibody—normal*
- *Saccharomyces cerevisiae antibodies (ASCA) (IGA, IGG)— positive for IGG and IGA antibodies*

All of Amber's tests were normal except for the saccharomyces cerevisiae antibodies. These antibodies are found in about 75 percent of patients with Crohn's disease. So Amber received the devastating news that she may have this chronic inflammatory disease of the intestines.

To verify Amber's Crohn's disease diagnosis, the gastroenterologist ordered more tests and obtained these results:

- *Stool test—negative*
- *X-ray of GI tract with color—negative*
- *Endoscopy with biopsy—negative*
- *Colonoscopy—negative*
- *CAT scan—negative*

Negative results on all of her secondary tests ruled out Crohn's disease. Instead, Amber was diagnosed with NCGS (non-celiac gluten sensitivity). Amber and her family were relieved because NCGS was not as severe and debilitating as Crohn's. Her GI issues improved through eating a gluten-free diet. Amber knows when she inadvertently eats foods containing gluten because her symptoms reoccur. However, she finds it challenging to figure out which foods contain hidden sources of gluten.

The lengthy list of symptoms for celiac disease and non-celiac gluten sensitivity involves numerous body systems. Surprisingly, more patients with gluten-related disorders present with nongastrointestinal symptoms, making it more challenging to diagnose. This chapter reviews the clinical tests available to diagnose these conditions.

After reading the multitude of symptoms and completing the symptom checklist associated with each gluten disorder in chapter 2, you should know whether you need testing. If your symptoms cause you to be concerned, talk with your physician. A gastroenterologist is likely more familiar with these disorders than your primary care physician.

If you currently eat a gluten-free diet, you should consume gluten daily for several weeks before being tested. Otherwise, the results may be false-negative because after a month of not eating gluten, your body no longer produces antibodies to fight it. An antibody is a blood protein the body creates to defend itself from a harmful invader— gluten. Many of these tests measure elevated levels of antibodies.

Unfortunately, not all medical personnel know that it is necessary for a patient to eat gluten weeks before testing. My daughter's physician emailed her the lab requisition for the antibody blood test. The nurse called to explain the test but failed to tell her she should eat foods with gluten to ensure accurate results. Since non-celiac gluten sensitivity is a new diagnosis (2010), not all medical staff have received thorough training about this condition and its appropriate diagnostic standards. That's why we must be informed patients.

Celiac Disease Testing

The following terminology gets a little confusing. The test names and terms like *antibodies* may be unfamiliar to you, so knowing what they are will be helpful. Usually, the diagnostic process starts with a physician ordering blood tests that check for gluten-related antibodies. If the initial tests are negative, your doctor will decide whether to order additional tests. When laboratory tests identify antibodies, the next step is usually a biopsy of the small intestine.

Blood Tests

Tissue Transglutaminase Antibody (tTG-IgA)

The most common and simplest test to diagnose celiac disease is tissue transglutaminase. If your body responds to the protein in gluten, it will create tTG enzymes measured in this test. This test is specific for CD. It will be positive in about 98 percent of individuals with CD who eat gluten. It will be positive in only about 5 percent of people who do not have CD.

A positive test indicates that the body identified gluten as an enemy and created antibodies as an immune response. If the test is positive, you probably have CD.

If this test is negative and your symptoms are minimal, your doctor may stop testing at this point. If further reasoning supports your belief that you may have CD, your doctor may order a second blood test to rule out an IgA deficiency. A small percentage of people do not produce the IgA antibody. People with celiac disease are more likely to experience an IgA deficiency. To rule out this deficiency, your doctor would order a total immunoglobulins (IgA) blood test. My daughter's doctor ordered both of the tests at the same time so she only needed one blood draw.

Total Immunoglobulins (IgA)

This test detects an IgA deficiency and verifies that your IgA levels are normal. If your IgA level is abnormally low, your tissue transglutaminase and endomysial antibody test may be false-negative. Therefore, you should have the gliadin antibody (deamidated) test.

Endomysial Antibody (EMA-IgA)

This test is more expensive, time-consuming, and difficult to process, so it is usually reserved for hard-to-diagnose patients. For example, if your tissue transglutaminase antibody test is negative or if a small intestine biopsy cannot be performed, then the endomysial antibody test may be ordered. This antibody test is specific for CD, but about 5–10 percent of individuals with CD have a false-negative result. If you tested positive for both tissue transglutaminase and endomysial antibody tests, it is extremely likely you have CD.

Gliadin Antibody Deamidated (IgA and IgG)

This fairly new test is used if an IgA deficiency is suspected or the tissue transglutaminase or endomysial antibody tests are negative. It looks for the level of gliadin (wheat protein) antibodies in your blood. More than 90 percent of people with CD or gluten sensitivity have higher-than-normal levels of this antibody, but few people without the disease do. A positive result may indicate gluten sensitivity and not CD. Further testing is needed to differentiate between the two diagnoses.

This test can also be used to check to see if a person with CD consumed hidden sources of gluten while on a gluten-free (GF) diet. It is more accurate with children and toddlers than the previously mentioned tests. Therefore, Tonya's (chapter 2 story) preschool-age children were tested for CD using this test. Even though Tonya's family ate a GF diet, she fed her children foods that contained gluten before being tested, as recommended by her doctor. One child tested positive for the disease, and the other did not.

Amber's doctor initially ordered both the tissue transglutaminase antibody and gliadin antibody (deamidated) tests. Both were negative. So the physician performed another blood test (saccharomyces cerevisiae antibodies) to rule out Crohn's disease. The result was positive. At that point in the diagnostic process, Amber thought she had Crohn's disease. With inconclusive results such as these, the next step was to perform a small intestine biopsy.

Additional Tests

Your physician may check for nutritional deficiencies and other abnormalities through the following tests:

- Vitamin B_{12}
- Vitamin D
- Complete blood count (CBC) tests for anemia and vitamin/mineral deficiencies
- Comprehensive metabolic panel to determine the status of kidney and liver functions as well as electrolyte, protein, and mineral levels
- C-reactive protein, which detects inflammation in the body
- While not a blood test, your physician may order a bone density test if you ever suffered from broken bones. When you do not absorb essential minerals, the thickness of your bones may be abnormally low.

Amber's doctor ordered a complete blood count, comprehensive metabolic panel, vitamin B_{12}, C-reactive protein, and H-pylori antibody test. (The bacteria H-pylori causes peptic ulcers.) Her vitamin B_{12} level was on the low side of normal so she would benefit from taking this supplement. All of the rest of her test results were normal.

At-Home Test Kit

A blood test you can perform at home, without a physician's order, is available at imaware™ (imaware.health/celiac-disease/at-home-blood-test/). This kit tests for tissue transglutaminase antibody and deamidated gliadin peptide—the same antibody tests Amber's gastroenterologist ordered. You obtain a blood sample through a small finger prick and collect five drops of blood into a microtube. Ship the sample to imaware™, and you receive the results online in about a week. This test is convenient and reasonably priced.

Genetic Tests

Genetic Test for Human Leukocyte Antigen—HLA–DQ2 and HLA–DQ8

Genetic testing has become a routine part of diagnosing celiac disease. Most people who have CD carry one or both of the human leukocyte antigen genes, but so do up to 30 percent of the population. Blood, saliva, or cheek swab genetic tests are available. The company 23andMe (Blog.23andme.com/health-traits/new-23andme-report-celiac-disease/) has an at-home celiac disease genetic test.

If you eat a GF diet and do not want to reintroduce gluten back into your diet because of its undesirable effects, you may choose to perform a genetic test before further invasive testing. Your diet does not influence genetic testing. It is the only test that does not require you to eat gluten at the time of testing. If you test negative for the CD gene, you have a 99 percent probability you will not get the disease, and no more testing is required. However, you could have non-celiac gluten sensitivity or wheat sensitivity.

You might never develop the disease if you tested positive for the CD gene, but you should have periodic testing performed if symptoms develop. As indicated previously, only 3 percent of individuals who carry the gene develop CD.

Since CD runs in families, if you tested positive for it, other members of your family should be screened for the disease. Individuals with a first-degree relative (child, parent, sibling) with CD have a 10 percent chance of developing the disease.[1] Celiac disease can develop at any age. Therefore, it is vital that first-degree relatives of someone with CD pursue genetic testing. If you carry the CD gene, screening for CD is recommended every three to five years.

Even if you don't have a relative with CD, you may want to pursue genetic testing if you had:

- Ambiguous antibody testing or intestinal biopsy results
- A discrepancy between the antibody tests and biopsy findings
- An unclear diagnosis of CD

I met a woman at a conference who had both a daughter and mother diagnosed with celiac disease. Yet she had never requested testing. After reviewing the symptoms listed in chapter 2, she realized she might have CD too since she suffered from Sjogren's disease (an autoimmune disorder) and many of the CD symptoms. After returning home, she tested positive for celiac disease. Now she understands why she suffered from many other ailments and the importance of following a strict GF diet.

Stool Tests

Your doctor may order a stool test. A sample of your stool is analyzed to determine if gluten-related antibodies exist. Amber's doctor ordered a stool test. The results were negative—no antibodies detected.

My daughter's (see chapter 4 story) stool test was positive for gluten antibodies. Her practitioner used the GI Microbial Assay Plus (GI-Map) DNA stool analysis by Quantitative PCR. This test provides a snapshot of the person's microbiome of the GI tract to determine whether it is healthy or imbalanced. This is a very important test as most of us have an imbalance of the beneficial versus harmful microbes in our gut. My daughter's blood tests were negative, so a NCGS diagnosis was determined through this test. Home testing stool kits are available through EnteroLab.

Diagnostic Process Next Steps

Negative blood, stool, and genetic tests mean the results are normal—you do not carry the CD gene or have gluten antibodies. A positive blood test indicates that further testing is needed. Your physician will reviews your test results, as well as your symptoms and medical history, to determine the next steps in the diagnostic process. Since Amber's symptoms were similar to Crohn's disease, her physician ordered additional testing to rule out this diagnosis.

Endoscopy

Small Intestine Biopsy

If blood tests were negative but your symptoms were highly indicative of celiac disease (like Amber's), your doctor may proceed with an intestinal biopsy. If a positive blood test indicates you might have CD, your doctor would confirm the diagnosis through a biopsy of the small intestine. During an endoscopy several biopsies (clipped samples of the villi) are taken from different areas in the small intestine.

Since damage to the villi occurs in patches, the samples obtained may not contain the harmed tissue, and the results could be false-negative. A literature review performed by the Oslo task force found that one biopsy confirmed the diagnosis of CD in two-thirds of patients and multiple biopsies confirmed CD in 95 percent. Unfortunately, diagnostic testing for CD is not a perfect science.

Marsh Classification

After the endoscopy, a pathologist will review the tissue samples under a microscope to determine if gluten-related damage exists. In 1992 Dr. Michael Marsh developed a classification system for the damaged villi—stages 1–4. Later Dr. Georg Oberhuber modified the Marsh Classification into five stages (1, 2, 3a, 3b, and 3c).[2] Don't you love the confusion?

Stage 1 means the intestinal lining is normal but immune cells are present. Immune cells are ready to engage in battle against what the body perceives as an enemy—gluten. Stage 3c (for the modified classification) or 4 (for the original Marsh classification) means the villi are entirely atrophied or flattened. Tonya's biopsy showed stage 4 CD with the original Marsh rating system, which was in use at that time. Amber's endoscopy and biopsy revealed one ulcer, but her villi were normal.

Celiac Disease Diagnostic Model

Since the diagnosis of CD can be quite complex, in 2010 a diagnostic model that includes a four-out-of-five rule became available.[3] A patient must exhibit four of the following indicators for a CD diagnosis:

1. Positive typical symptoms for CD
2. Positive blood tests for CD, including tissue transglutaminase or endomysial antibody
3. Positive genetic testing for human leukocyte antigen HLA-DQ2 or HLA-DQ8 genes
4. Positive small intestine biopsy showing damaged villi

5. Improvement of symptoms with a GF diet

If you plan to pursue testing, educate yourself about the diagnostic process to help solve your gluten puzzle. Understanding this four-out-of-five rule will ensure you have all of these indicators checked. Ultimately, your goal is a firm diagnosis, relief of symptoms, and a plan to heal so you can live a healthier life.

Interpreting Test Results

As you can see from the multitude of tests, CD testing is multifaceted. You almost need an if-then diagram to determine the next step. My sister did not get tested until after she had removed gluten from her diet. Therefore, her blood tests and small intestine biopsy results were negative. Thankfully, the intestinal lining begins to heal as soon as an individual stops eating gluten—a testament to how quickly the body heals itself.

Non-Celiac Gluten Sensitivity Testing

Surprisingly, a specific test to diagnose NCGS does not exist. Blood tests identify signs of NCGS such as anemia, high liver enzymes, and low potassium levels. If you test negative for CD, and your symptoms resolve through eating a GF diet, you most likely have NCGS. Recently, researchers agreed on a set of factors an individual must meet for a NCGS diagnosis:

1. Negative celiac panel blood tests
2. Negative small intestine biopsy
3. Symptoms improve when gluten is eliminated
4. No other medical explanation for symptoms

Amber met all four of the criteria listed. Therefore, she was diagnosed with NCGS and not Crohn's disease. If you experience symptoms of a gluten-related illness that your physician has not diagnosed, ruling out NCGS is essential. Eliminating gluten from your diet becomes the next logical step.

Both gluten sensitivity and irritable bowel syndrome (IBS) are diagnosed through ruling out other disorders. So if you have been diagnosed with IBS, it could actually be gluten sensitivity. There is no specific test for IBS or gluten sensitivity.

Wheat Sensitivity Testing

The muddled middle ground between NCGS and a wheat allergy is wheat sensitivity or intolerance. I am wheat sensitive, so my body does not react well when I eat foods containing wheat. So I avoid wheat.

In chapter 2, we discussed the difference between gluten sensitivity and wheat sensitivity. Someone can differentiate whether they are sensitive to wheat or gluten by the following process:

1. Eat a GF diet for a month until you no longer experience symptoms.
2. After a month, add back food items made with barley or rye to see if you develop adverse effects.

Purchase pearled barley from your local health food store. It tastes, looks, and cooks similar to brown rice. Barley is not wheat. If you do not experience symptoms after consuming it, you may be wheat sensitive and not gluten sensitive—like me. You might be able to eat gluten in a nonwheat form.

Wheat Allergy Testing

The body does not develop an allergy to gluten, per se, but can be allergic to wheat, rye, and/or barley. Wheat is one of the most common allergens and the body's reaction may be similar to other food allergies such as shellfish. If you are allergic to a food, you should avoid eating it so you don't suffer from allergic symptoms.

If you appear to have an allergy, your doctor may refer you to an allergist or immunologist for testing. A skin test is the most common type of allergy testing. However, blood tests can verify a food allergy too. The two types of allergy testing include:

- Skin prick tests—the patient's skin is pricked with a needle that contains a tiny amount of an allergen. The nurse documents the reaction by measuring the size and elevation of a welt that develops. If no skin reaction occurs, the patient is not allergic to the allergen.
- Blood tests—measure the amount of allergen-specific antibodies for a food or substance.

I received a wheat allergy diagnosis through a skin prick test on my back at age ten. A skin prick test is unpleasant but tolerable—unless you ask my daughter. She reacted to thirty-two of forty-eight allergens and fainted during the procedure. Thankfully, I caught her before she fell off the examining table! No gluten-related disorder or testing is for the faint of heart.

Summary

Information about testing for a gluten disorder is the next step to solving your diagnostic puzzle. Unfortunately, no single test—blood test, genetic test, or intestinal biopsy—can diagnose a gluten-related disorder. Instead, it is the combination of the patient's symptoms, testing results, and response to a GF diet that leads to a diagnosis.

If your diagnosis is inconclusive, you might want to be tested again at a later time. Despite negative test results, you can still develop CD in the future, at any age. As previously mentioned, celiac disease needs three conditions to develop—genetic predisposition, consumption of gluten, and an environmental trigger. If I carried the CD gene, I would remove gluten from my diet to prevent celiac disease from developing.

The symptoms of CD mimic other conditions, including irritable bowel syndrome. Doctors may not think of CD when a patient presents with nongastrointestinal symptoms, so they don't test for it. However, a patient must diligently work to obtain a diagnosis before irreparable damage occurs (like Tonya).

Sadly, most people who have CD remain undiagnosed. Many people diagnosed with a gluten-related condition reported a long-standing history of symptoms that should have raised suspicion long before their health declined to the point of debilitating symptoms. Hopefully, in the future it won't take as long to obtain a diagnosis. It only took four months for Amber's gastroenterologist to determine her diagnosis.

GLUTEN-RELATED DISORDERS: TREATMENT AND TRANSITION

Sarah's Story

In intermediate school, my daughter Sarah experienced headaches. Her doctor referred her to an optometrist, who prescribed glasses, not for her vision (20/20) but to prevent overfocusing. The glasses did not help. She continued to suffer from headaches throughout high school.

Sarah suffered from exhaustion during her senior year. Her doctor ordered a complete blood count (CBC), but the results showed normal levels. She left for college a few months later.

During her first semester away, she prepared most of her meals. However, the following semester, she primarily ate out. She became alarmed when she experienced nosebleeds for the first time in her life.

In May of that year, Sarah was prescribed an antibiotic for a urinary tract infection. In August, she traveled to Europe for three weeks. Upon returning to college in the fall, she experienced constant exhaustion, hair loss, and digestive issues (gas, gurgling, diarrhea).

While at home for Christmas break, Sarah wanted to see her doctor but found no openings. So a reputable, local clinician performed iridology, the practice of diagnosing health issues by examining the iris of the eye. The results were low magnesium, adrenal fatigue, anxiety, aggravated pancreas, low functioning liver, bloating, and gas. She started taking adrenal fatigue *vitamins and magnesium. After several months on these supplements, she regained some energy.*

By May of her sophomore year, she became irritable and moody. She also suffered from acne, disturbed sleep, and more severe digestive issues (gas, frequent diarrhea, burping). Her doctor ordered laboratory tests that revealed a deficiency in vitamin B_{12} and adrenal fatigue. He prescribed vitamin B_{12} shots, adrenal fatigue vitamins twice daily, magnesium to improve sleep, L-glutamine (a supplement that supports intestinal health), and probiotics to improve gut health.

By the summer, Sarah's sleep and moodiness improved. However, her digestive issues and acne persisted. In the fall of her junior year, her gastrointestinal symptoms worsened. After every meal, she experienced immediate bloating and gas within thirty minutes, followed by burping and sometimes diarrhea. Most days after dinner, and into the following morning, she experienced diarrhea—up to four episodes every night. Sarah's roller-coaster digestive health ruled her life. Desperate for an improvement in her health, she tried a gluten-free diet for three weeks before Thanksgiving, which decreased her diarrhea and gas.

At Thanksgiving she ate gluten again, and her digestive symptoms worsened. She felt tired, her acne worsened, and she was ill for weeks. While on Christmas break, she talked to her Aunt Ginny, my sister (see her story in chapter 5), who is highly gluten sensitive. After their conversation, Sarah suspected she might be gluten sensitive too. For the next three weeks, she ate a gluten-free diet, and her diarrhea lessened. She also started taking digestive enzymes per Ginny's suggestion.

She began to evaluate everything she ate. In January, Sarah found that onions and garlic caused digestive issues, so she stopped using them. Ginny warned her that many spices contain gluten, so Sarah purchased gluten-free spices and began cooking more for herself. She continued to seek out the cause of her consistent gas, belching, and diarrhea.

Parties with friends were the worst. Most party foods are loaded with gluten. I suggested she take a gluten/dairy-free pizza to parties. The pizza chain Mellow Mushroom makes delicious gluten-free pizzas and is diligent in avoiding cross-contamination with gluten-free foods.

On a visit home, Sarah asked her doctor to order a gluten sensitivity test.

He ordered the gliadin antibody (deamidated) blood test (IgA and IgG). The staff at the doctor's office failed to tell her that she needed to be eating gluten for the test to be valid, but I did.

Before she had the test, Sarah started a two-week gluten challenge where she ate about two pieces of bread per day. During the challenge, her cheeks became rounder and fuller (swollen). She realized for the first time that she'd had puffy cheeks her whole life. Her acne worsened and her nosebleeds returned, accompanied by gas, bloating, and more frequent loose stools. Her test results were negative. She was not gluten sensitive. She slowly incorporated gluten back into her diet. The same symptoms that got worse when she did the challenge continued.

Next, her doctor ordered a food sensitivity blood test. The results showed Sarah was highly sensitivity to soybeans and moderately sensitive to apples, corn, cow's milk, barley, yeast, and egg whites. She was diagnosed with leaky gut syndrome (also called impaired intestinal permeability). To heal her GI tract, she was prescribed L-glutamine and digestive enzymes supplements, which she was already taking.

Over the summer and fall, Sarah continued to experience digestive problems despite taking supplements and avoiding everything identified as sensitive for her. Other foods like onions, garlic, and sweet potatoes irritated her gut even though she was not sensitive to them. Sometimes she suffered from painful stomachaches after eating her own carefully prepared dinner. After years of working with her physician with no resolution to her problems, she found a holistic practitioner. The nurse practitioner ordered a stool test to check for parasites, an imbalance of the gut flora, gluten sensitivity, and Candida.

The test revealed that her stools contained gluten antibodies. She was gluten sensitive after all! Also, higher than normal levels of Candida were present, and the beneficial probiotics that she got from food, not supplements, were low. The nurse practitioner prescribed a gluten-free, autoimmune diet along with L-glutamine to heal her leaky gut. Sarah also followed the recommendation of three months of a Biocidin Candida cleanse .

Within two months, Sarah's bloating, gas, and diarrhea went away. Now when she experiences GI symptoms, she knows she accidentally ate gluten.

Today, she rarely suffers from headaches or nosebleeds. Her health puzzle was finally solved.

In the past three chapters, you learned about the four types of gluten-related disorders, their symptoms (symptom checklist in chapter 2), and diagnostic tests. Now we will discuss the only treatment for all gluten-related disorders—eating a wheat-free or gluten-free diet. A transition to this new lifestyle includes many emotional, social, physical, and mental adjustments. This chapter will help you make those changes smoothly.

Gluten and wheat sensitivity are challenging to diagnose. Obtaining an accurate diagnosis takes time, patience, and money. Sometimes many tests are needed to figure out the puzzle. It is frustrating and disheartening to continue to suffer from digestive and health issues and remain unable to determine the cause.

If you are experiencing such frustration with undiagnosed symptoms, be diligent in working with your healthcare practitioner until you are satisfied with the results. My daughter Sarah almost gave up, but she tried one last holistic practitioner—a functional medicine advanced registered nurse practitioner. Finally, her gluten puzzle was solved. If you have come to a roadblock and are still without a diagnosis, change doctors or try a gluten-free (GF) diet, but do not give up until your puzzle is solved.

If you have celiac disease or gluten sensitivity, the treatment is following a strict GF diet. For wheat sensitivity and wheat allergy, remove all sources of wheat from your diet. It takes time and guidance to learn how to make these dietary changes. Chapter 6 provides you with the nutritional support you need.

Adjustment Phase

If you have been diagnosed with a gluten-related disorder, you need to work through an emotional roller coaster. After the shock wears off, you may experience anger and then sadness as you grieve the loss of gluten. These comfort foods include many family favorites such as chicken and dumplings and apple pie. These feelings are normal. Allow yourself time to process them.

You may fear letting go of your favorite foods, being deprived and different, or having to eat flavorless food. Stomp out your fears. Try new dishes. Realize that the old gluten-containing foods made you feel sick. You will discover new comfort foods. I did. Gluten-free dishes don't have to deprive you of flavor. Many taste fabulous, improve your health, and give you energy. Who doesn't want those results?

Don't dwell on the negative aspects of this new lifestyle. That's not healthy either. Besides, no one wants to be around someone who is self-pitying. After you have processed your emotions, move on. Embrace the GF lifestyle with a positive attitude.

Emotional Impact

You may experience mixed emotions in adjusting to a GF diet—from elation to devastation. Glad to finally figure out the root cause of your health issues, but also grieving the loss of your favorite foods.

My daughter Sarah experienced difficulty coming to terms with her diagnosis. She felt upset and relieved simultaneously. She was thankful to know if she stopped eating gluten, her leaky gut and food sensitivities would heal, and her digestive issues would subside. However, she knew the transition would be difficult.

What feelings might you be experiencing? Journaling is therapeutic. I wrote *Healthy Living Journal* to help others make and maintain necessary lifestyle changes for a healthier future. This book provides space for journaling along the journey of transition. I encourage you to write down the feelings you experience as you switch to a GF life. This will help you navigate the ups and downs.

A sense of loss at not being able to eat some of your favorite foods is normal. Eating a GF diet is a lifelong treatment and commitment. I sometimes feel I am missing out on a treat when I go to an Italian restaurant and can't eat the bread dipped in the herb oil, nor enjoy my favorite dessert, tiramisu. Feeling depressed about this change is natural. Allow yourself time to mourn the loss. But the benefits of eating GF outweigh the loss.

Take a look at the symptoms you experience from the chapter 2 checklist. Think about those symptoms diminishing. The changes in your eating habits are a journey so you can live an abundant life, not a life filled with disease and unwanted, unhealthy symptoms. When you take the steps outlined in this book, your health and energy levels improve because you eat GF foods that nourish your body.

Do you fear that you can't make the necessary diet modifications? Poor eating habits are hard to break. Some causes of dysfunctional eating habits include an emotional association with food, a food addiction, or Candida overgrowth in the GI tract. My faith-based book 7 Steps to Get Off Sugar and Carbohydrates helps people find the root cause of inappropriate eating habits and succeed in changing their lifestyle. Feel free to join my private Facebook group 7 Steps to Get Off Sugar and Carbohydrates. Through this group, I am available to answer your questions and provide you with encouragement and support you may need.

Do you have an emotional connection to certain foods that you can't break on your own? If so, you may benefit from my book *Christian Study Guide for 7 Steps to Get Off Sugar and Carbohydrates,* which can help you break the chains of food addiction, once and for all.

Since there is no treatment for gluten-related disorders other than a GF or wheat-free diet, my daughter felt she had no choice but to eat GF. She wanted her symptoms and food sensitivities to go away. Even though she knew a dietary change was the treatment that would heal her and give her a more satisfying life, it was a difficult decision. She needed resolve. Deciding is the challenging first step toward making this lifestyle change.

Periodically you may need to return to your original decision and recommit to it as situations (vacations, weddings, and parties) or temptations challenge your palate. Stand firm in your decision to eat GF foods, even when you falter. It is hard to be perfect. So aim for consistency, remain steadfast, and committed.

Social Adjustment

Eating GF can feel stressful and isolating. It requires knowledge plus trial-and-error to discern what foods contain gluten. Socializing becomes more difficult. What will you order at a restaurant? Will you find something to eat at the potluck dinner? These situations can cause anxiety. Chapter 7 will help you navigate each eating menu.

Simply explain to close friends and family that you have a gluten-related diagnosis and require a GF diet. Advise them that you would appreciate their willingness to offer food choices to accommodate you whenever you are sharing a home-cooked meal together. Most people are happy to make small menu changes for those they love and care about especially if given a few simple menu ideas.

I appreciate others' willingness to add a couple of GF dishes to a meal when I'm joining them. I always express my gratitude. My family and close friends want me to be healthy. I can eat fresh fruits, vegetables, and meats if they don't have a sauce or spice that contains gluten. I offer to bring a dish or two to shared meals. At a potluck meal, I usually don't have a problem choosing GF items because of the large selection generally available. I typically select fresh produce, nuts, and a slice of meat, in addition to the GF dish I brought myself.

Maintaining a GF diet can be quite intimidating since the burden of your success is based on how well you make consistent choices—especially when you didn't know Aunt Sally's casserole contained gluten. You'll have a learning curve with this new lifestyle. You'll make mistakes and feel the consequences. Yet as you gain knowledge, your confidence will increase. With time, the new diet will become second nature. A year from now, your outlook will be better. Give yourself grace.

It is human nature to want what we can't have. However, focusing on what you can eat, rather than what you cannot eat, promotes a positive attitude. To assist you with making this transition, create a list of the positive benefits of adopting a gluten-free regime. Tell others how great you feel and how this diet is helping you improve your health. Instead of grieving over the loss of your gluten-free foods, be joyous about your improved health.

After my daughter had time to adjust to her diagnosis, she decided to embrace a GF lifestyle with a positive attitude. She became excited about the new diet and ordered a GF cookbook (appendix 3 includes fifty GF recipes). She studied the dietary handouts the nurse practitioner gave her to get started, including a list of foods she could and couldn't eat, which helped her plan menus (see chapter 6 for menu planning).

Surgery, drugs, and treatments are not needed to treat these gluten-related disorders. Instead, relief comes from dietary modification. As the body heals, many symptoms lessen or diminish altogether. With celiac disease, the villi heal if you are diagnosed early and adhere to a strict GF eating plan.

I have been wheat-free for eight years now, and I feel immeasurably better. I experience bountiful energy and clarity of mind. Cute outfits fit me once again. Writing, traveling, and exercising is no longer demanding. I live a joyful life with overwhelming motivation. I hope you begin to experience a more abundant life too!

Physical Effect

Our bodies are designed to heal themselves naturally. One year after Amber (chapter 3) embraced a gluten-free lifestyle she writes, "My health has definitely improved! My migraines have completely stopped (before I suffered from one almost every day). I gained twenty pounds, which is definitely a good thing, and I have regular solid bowel movements now."

Unfortunately, when we consume food our body is sensitive or allergic to, it causes inflammation. Medical practitioners now point to inflammation as the root of most diseases. Though our bodies can and do heal themselves, like Amber's, when invasion from inflammation causes physical problems, we need to help our bodies get on the right path toward recovery.

With a gluten-related disorder, the gastrointestinal tract becomes inflamed and possibly damaged. Openings in the bowel walls, known as leaky gut or intestinal permeability, may develop. These holes allow harmful microorganisms and food particles to enter the bloodstream. Our bodies don't recognize these particles, so our immune system creates antibodies that cause food allergies and autoimmune diseases to develop.[1]

You can work on healing your gut by eating more vegetables, fruits, non-gluten grains, nuts, seeds, and meat. Bone broth is healing for the GI tract. Avoid processed foods contained in boxes and bags that have a long shelf life—which indicates the presence of unhealthy preservatives. A daily probiotic with at least ten strains of beneficial microorganisms may benefit your GI tract. You can choose to take a probiotic for a couple of months or long term. Eat foods rich in beneficial probiotics such as kimchi, sauerkraut, and cultured foods like plain Greek yogurt. You can't get all the beneficial GI bacteria from a supplement. Some must come from foods.

In addition to leaky gut, the GI tract may not be able to absorb vitamins and minerals from food when it is irritated and inflamed. When foods can't be adequately absorbed, malnutrition sets in. Some individuals with CD have voracious appetites because their bodies don't absorb the nutrients in food. They lack essential vitamins, minerals, and omega-three oils, so they crave more food to gain needed nourishment. Some may even become obese yet still be malnourished. After an individual stops consuming gluten, her body heals, and she can once again absorb nutrients from food.

Consuming a lot of foods derived from white flour keeps the body from receiving the necessary vitamins and minerals it needs. White flour is among the most prevalent wheat products used today. A wheat berry consists of three layers: bran, germ, and endosperm. White flour contains one part of the wheat kernel—the endosperm, which is mostly starch. The other two parts of wheat contain the fiber and nutrients. These are not included in white flour. This type of flour has been chemically bleached, consequently, the grain no longer resembles the wholesome food it once was.

Once Sarah began eating a GF diet, she was ravenous. For six weeks, she consumed larger than normal portions and ate more frequently. Her previous diet had been deficient in essential nutrients. In the beginning she fought food cravings. But once she stopped eating wheat, her body began to crave wholesome foods with essential vitamins, minerals, and protein.

When one removes the substance causing the inflammation, the body heals. It takes time and adherence to a strict diet to see the benefits. However, once you get past the first month or two, the decrease in symptoms outweighs the loss of gluten-laden foods. So don't give up too early.

As my daughter transitioned to a healthy GF diet, she appeared to come out of a fog. Instead of being tired and nonconversational all the time, she became alert, happy, and a joy to be around. I got my daughter back because a nutrient-rich diet with more protein and omega-three oils provided the amino acids her brain needed to produce the neuro-stimulating hormones that improve mood.

You are on the verge of getting your life back too. A common gluten-related symptom is fatigue—a chronic type of exhaustion that leaves you weak. I experienced fatigue for years until I changed my diet. You may not have the stamina or desire to perform normal activities, like cooking or cleaning.

Fatigue can be caused by your body not absorbing nutrients. Once you change your diet, the inflammation in your small intestine will resolve, and your body will absorb nutrients again. Then your fatigue and other symptoms will go away. Chapters 5 and 6 will help guide you through the transition to a GF eating plan.

. . .

Mental Impact

Depression and anxiety continue to increase in our culture at alarming rates. Could there be a correlation between our grain-based (mostly wheat) modern diet and these escalating mental health issues? The brain needs amino acids to produce mood-enhancing chemicals such as serotonin. White flour is devoid of these amino acids.

When people with gluten-related disorders consume gluten, they can develop depression, anxiety, and mood swings. Medical studies show that eliminating gluten reduces depression for such individuals.[2] When you stop eating gluten, similar symptoms may resolve.

These mental conditions affect relationships and the ability to enjoy life. Heather (see chapter 7 story) had such negative psychological symptoms from consuming gluten that she became depressed. Once she was diagnosed and began a GF diet, her depression subsided. She eventually opened several successful GF restaurants. Merely altering her diet improved her mental wellness and led to a new dream. A sense of well-being is one of the many benefits of a GF lifestyle.

Family Adjustment

A family member with a gluten-related ailment affects the whole family. Just as it takes time for you to come to terms with this diagnosis and its lifelong dietary modification, your loved ones will need an adjustment period too. Seek to work through this adjustment together.

A typical response is denial. One family member may not believe eating one breadcrumb could affect you negatively. Other family members want to know how this will impact them. Will they have to change their diet too? Can they continue to eat pasta and bread?

Everyone needs to process his or her emotions. If you or a family member experience resentment or anger, acknowledge those feelings and express them without judgment. Time and understanding help as you work through these emotions and share them with each other.

As you learn more about your disorder, educate your family. The more they know, the better. They will most likely run across numerous other people in their lives who have a gluten-related condition, since 10 percent of the nation's population is now affected. As you share your challenge with your family, they may become more sympathetic with others who have similar ailments. Compassion and understanding are crucial. You might be surprised how supportive some family members and friends can be to your diagnosis.

Will the whole family have to eat a GF diet? Not necessarily, however, if the entire family eats GF, there is no risk of cross-contamination. Plus you only need to cook one version of a meal. But lack of choice may create bitterness with some. Some families compromise; most meals will be GF, but some favorite pasta or gluten-related dish will be served occasionally. Find what works best for your family.

Since I am the cook, I continue to provide my family with pasta made from wheat, but I also serve spaghetti squash. I serve a gluten and non-gluten form of many foods. I also provide a couple of different vegetables. The whole family appreciates that they can choose what they like. When you are GF, meal planning and preparation are essential. We will address this in chapter 6.

Adjustment to a Child's Diagnosis

It can be shocking to find out your child has a gluten-related ailment. You anticipated a perfectly healthy kid, but he cannot tolerate gluten or wheat. You may experience a period of grieving. However, you will quickly realize this diagnosis is harder on you than it is on your child.

The good news is that your kid can be happy, healthy, and gluten-free. Your child does not have cancer, nor need surgery or medication. Your attitude can influence how he feels about his gluten-related disorder. Therefore, take time to adjust slowly so you can be sure your approach is positive. Listening ears hear what you tell others about their condition. Children are more flexible and resilient than you think. Your youngster is probably more concerned about his next ballgame than his diet. You will likely be more affected emotionally by the diagnosis than your child.

To promote a positive attitude, provide your son or daughter with specific examples of how life will be better with a GF diet. Many physical or behavioral problems improve. Attention deficit disorder or attention deficit hyperactivity disorder may decrease or go away completely.[3] Wouldn't it be wonderful not to medicate your kid for these disorders?

No matter the age of your child who is diagnosed with a gluten disorder, you will want to educate him. Age-appropriate books are available to teach children and teens about their disorder. Some are even picture books for younger ones. Ask your local librarian or bookstore staff, or search for appropriate books online.

If your child can read, teach her to read food labels. Involve her in planning the weekly menu, including making lunch for school. Have her accompany you to the supermarket with your grocery list. Try to make it fun.

Involve your kid in the kitchen by creating delicious snacks, meals, and desserts. Help her experience how GF foods can be just as tasty and more nutritional than foods containing gluten. Teach her about the nutrients contained in these foods.

Always have appropriate snacks available at home, school, and sporting events. Packing a bag of nuts or trail mix can be a lifesaver. When your youth desires a food containing gluten, always be prepared with a healthy gluten-free substitute. If you have a delicious snack readily available, it will make life easier. You may want to bring a GF dessert for your child to restaurants if other family members will be ordering dessert.

Ordering food at restaurants provides the perfect opportunity to train your youngster to determine which items on the menu are GF. Demonstrate how to ask the server questions about the menu, and your child will also learn to be assertive. Today, most restaurants serve GF options.

At birthday parties and holidays, your child may feel as though she doesn't fit in because she can't eat birthday cake or holiday foods.

Contact the person in charge of an event ahead of time and offer to provide delicious GF options. You will expand your culinary talent and help your child and others enjoy healthier food options. With a positive attitude, cooking can be fun.

Help your kid overcome the embarrassment of being different by explaining that one out of every ten individuals has one of these disorders. Teach your children that many people have challenges, but some are more visible than others. Be perceptive and ready when teachable moments come along. When your child learns coping skills about her own health, she'll also develop compassion toward others who have similar disorders.

As children gain knowledge about their gluten-related diagnoses, they will be better able to articulate their needs to friends, family members, and other adults. Teach them to say "No, thank you," when offered food that may contain gluten. Saying no is better than risking the consequences.

If your child does ingest gluten, which will occur from time to time, help her understand why she feels ill. Her stomachache, diarrhea, or other symptoms are a direct result of eating gluten. When a kid understands this connection, she's much less likely to sneak unhealthy foods.

Many resources and support groups are available to assist you in dealing with a GF lifestyle for yourself or your child. You can find celiac disease support groups all across the US and a list of GF summer camps at ROCK Raising Our Celiac Kids. Appendix 2 lists additional resources.

The younger your child is when diagnosed, the easier the transition to a GF diet. It is more difficult to change a teenager's palate than a toddler's. As your adolescent grows, continue to have ongoing conversations about the GF lifestyle.

Your teenager must manage her GF diet once she leaves home, so trust her to make appropriate food choices when you see she is ready. If a mistake causes discomfort, she will realize the importance of paying better attention to her food selection.

In the adolescent years, certain symptoms may diminish. If this occurs, teens may be tempted to eat foods containing gluten. Yet as GI symptoms subside, more adult-like issues may evolve, such as headaches, fatigue, and depression instead of bloating, stomachaches, and diarrhea. Help your teenager understand that these new symptoms are also signs of gluten intolerance.

Even after your young adult leaves home, you can send her a care package with some of her favorite gluten-free snacks. Learning to make healthy choices is a recipe for success for any person. As a parent, it is an incredible responsibility and opportunity to teach your child to eat a nutritious GF diet so that she can live an abundant, healthy life.

Holistic Approach

Your body needs to heal from the damage caused by consuming gluten or wheat. Your body's reaction to this substance caused you to develop many symptoms you want to eliminate. A holistic approach to healing will speed your recovery.

If you need additional support making this lifestyle change, purchase my course, 7 Steps to Reclaim Your Health and Optimal Weight (https://susanuneal.com/courses/7-steps-to-get-off-sugar-and-carbs-course). In this course I walk you through the steps to change your eating habits once and for all.

In addition to making dietary changes, be sure to appropriately deal with stress, get adequate sleep, and perform gentle forms of exercise. Stress tends to cause people to crave carbohydrates, sugary comfort foods, and junk food. Processed foods give you a sugar rush, but when your blood sugar crashes, you feel rotten. This blood-sugar fluctuation leads to anxiety because your body has to secrete adrenaline to counteract the drop in blood sugar.

Determine the stressors (things that cause you stress) in your life, and list them in your journal. Can you do something about the stressors? Evaluate each one and brainstorm on how to minimize them. Ask your partner, family members, or friends for help in dealing with your stressors. Some need professional help to alleviate stress.

How do you cope with stress? Do you tend to deal with it through undesirable eating habits? If so, recognize this and choose to do something about your stress level. Can you eliminate a stressor in your life? Some stress-relieving activities include enjoying a massage, journaling, listening to soothing music, praying or meditating, and calling a friend.

Exercise is another positive coping strategy for dealing with stress. It burns off adrenaline and improves sleep. However, while your body is in the earlier stages of recovering from gluten-related symptoms, focus on gentle forms of exercise such as walking, swimming, or yoga.

It doesn't matter what type of gentle exercise you do as long as you do it. Take a group fitness class like Pilates or water aerobics. After you begin feeling better, try to increase exercise to at least twenty minutes three times a week.

In addition to physical exercise, yoga and meditation calm the mind and body. Mindfulness exercises train a person to pay attention to cravings or stressors without reacting to them. The idea is to ride out the wave of intense desire. As a person becomes more mindful, she may learn why she wants to indulge. Meditation quiets the part of the brain that can lead to loops of obsession. I've created several meditative yoga products including DVDs, books, and card decks available at Christianyoga.com.

Restful sleep is essential for well-being. We need at least eight hours per night for optimal brain health and prevention of dementia and Alzheimer's.[4] These brain diseases are on the rise, and most of us have a loved one or know someone who suffers from them. Sleep and diet affect the brain. If you sleep less than eight hours or eat unhealthy foods, you'll be affected physically and psychologically.

I stop drinking fluids at 6 pm so I don't have to go to the bathroom so often at night. Getting up in the middle of the night disrupts sleep. Plan when you will consume your eight glasses of water during the day, and avoid consuming a lot of water after dinner.

Not being able to eat gluten is a significant lifestyle change, but the payoff is phenomenal. This holistic approach will help your body heal faster. Be sure to document in your journal as each symptom subsides.

Summary

If you find yourself discouraged by your diagnosis, make a list in your journal of everything positive about your new lifestyle. For example, you will be eating a healthier diet, your body will heal, and your symptoms will go away. An attitude of gratitude changes a person's outlook for the better.

Remember that the GF diet gets easier with time. So does eating out at restaurants and social events. You may also enjoy a more positive outlook on life. Many individuals didn't realize how bad they felt until they began eating GF. Fortunately, much of the damage caused by eating gluten is reversible. After some time, the malnutrition and malabsorption issues, bone loss, achy joints, and many other symptoms resolve. Just like Amber's did. You were created to enjoy an abundant life, and you are well on your way to regaining your health.

5

EMBRACE THE GLUTEN-FREE LIFESTYLE

Ginny's Story

In her early 50s, my sister Ginny experienced unpleasant digestive issues. She noticed this usually occurred when she cooked homemade chicken potpie. The morning after eating the potpie, she suffered from multiple episodes of foul-smelling, floating stools.

She usually thought, "There must have been salmonella in the chicken, so I need to be more careful washing my hands when I cook."

She tried a probiotic (beneficial microorganism) supplement for her digestive tract, and at first it helped. A few years later, she developed gastroesophageal reflux. Her primary care physician prescribed Prilosec and digestive enzymes and suggested she try a gluten-free (GF) diet. She did for a few weeks. Unfortunately, her symptoms did not go away because she did not realize how many foods besides bread and pasta contain gluten.

One day a bout of diarrhea was so severe, she went to an urgent care center. While there, she shook so badly the doctor rushed her by ambulance to the hospital. She was admitted for a life-threatening low-potassium level and dehydration. The incident of low potassium left her with a condition where she got jittery and shook easily, so her doctor prescribed a beta-blocker (a cardiac medication) she took daily. She hated having to take medication and its side effects.

Later that year, she came to my house for Christmas. She told me about her GI symptoms. Intermittently, her chest burned like fire from reflux. Her abdominal pain felt like someone punched her in the stomach and she lay in bed with a heating pad over her abdomen for hours. A large volume of liquefied stools followed the excruciating abdominal pain. She also described having brain fog and trouble focusing.

When I heard about her severe symptoms, I suggested a GF diet to see if her symptoms improved. Ginny told me she'd tried a GF diet, but it made no difference. I encouraged her to try again because it takes time to figure out all the different foods that contain gluten.

After the holidays, she further investigated how to eat gluten-free on the website celiac.org (see appendix 2 for a list of resources). Three days after implementing the diet, her digestive symptoms resolved. Ginny felt significantly better—her brain fog vanished, and her attention deficit disorder calmed.

After eating GF for several months, her doctor ran blood tests for celiac disease, but they were negative. Once a person stops eating gluten, the body's reaction—creating gluten antibodies—ceases. Blood tests measure the number of gluten antibodies. Since her tests were negative, but her symptoms resolved with a GF diet, she was diagnosed with non-celiac gluten sensitivity. However, she could have CD and not know it because she was tested after removing gluten from her diet. Next, she plans to pursue genetic testing to see if she carries the celiac disease gene.

Maybe you or a loved one was diagnosed with a gluten-related disorder, or you decided to try a gluten-free diet. Individuals who follow a gluten-free diet without having celiac disease are referred to as a PWAG (people who avoid gluten).

At first, it feels overwhelming—even nearly impossible—to stop eating foods that contain gluten. However, after you've gotten the hang of it, this lifestyle will become second nature. This chapter will guide you as you transition to a gluten-free life.

One of the most overwhelming factors in moving to a GF diet is discovering that gluten is everywhere. It is found in thousands of food products, making the switch to GF difficult. Most people don't realize that even salad dressings contain gluten. Ginny did not attain relief the first time she tried to eat a gluten-free diet because she ingested gluten through hidden sources. When you transition to this new lifestyle, understanding how to do it correctly is vital.

Once Ginny stopped eating gluten, the nutritional value of her diet improved. She ate rich sources of protein from meat, fish, nuts, seeds, and beans. She cooked at least two fresh vegetables with each meal. To season foods she used only salt, pepper, fresh herbs, onions, garlic, and shallots. Therefore, she consumed more vitamins, minerals, and micronutrients that made her body function well.

Think of foods as being dead or alive. Food from a bag sitting on the shelf for months is dead and fails to give your body nutrients. On the other hand, fresh vegetables contain essential vitamins the body needs.

Avoid prepackaged, GF processed foods. Many contain rice flour and sugar, placing them high on the glycemic index. This index ranks foods on a scale of one to one hundred based on how they raise the blood-sugar level. These foodlike substances are frequently quick and easy to prepare, so it's tempting to try them. However, when we eat packaged foods—even those labeled gluten-free—we fill an immediate craving without thinking of the long-term consequences. In addition, packaged GF products may contain a little bit of gluten—20 parts per million is an acceptable standard for GF labeling. For those with CD or highly gluten sensitive individuals, like Ginny, eating these products may elicit symptoms.

Instead, replace processed products with whole, natural foods. An organic green apple costs less and contains more nutrition than a so-called GF item packaged in colorful, enticing boxes and bags. Fiber in fruit and vegetables fills your stomach and tells your body you are full. Processed foods remove the fiber so it takes a larger quantity of food to become full—so you eat more. The fiber in fruit slows digestion, which reduces the effects of sugar in raising your blood-sugar levels. As you eliminate processed foods from your diet, begin to consume more whole, organic fruits and vegetables; whole grains (brown rice, quinoa); beans; fish; meat; nuts; and seeds. Your body will thank you for nourishing it properly and respond by healing.

Each time you eat, look at your food and assess whether or not it is good for you. If a person primarily eats dead food, how does the body get the proper nutrients it needs? Improper nutrition causes cells in our bodies to get sick and mutate, and not function properly. When a cell within the human body replicates incorrectly, it becomes cancer. How can your body replace old cells with healthy new ones if you don't nourish it with the essential vitamins and minerals it requires? It can't.

Check labels and do not eat any foods containing wheat, gluten, barley, or rye. Also, to improve your health, try not to eat foods with more than five ingredients or more than 10 grams of sugar per serving. If you can't pronounce an ingredient, your body probably won't recognize it as food either. Begin to simplify your diet. For example, eat two hard-boiled eggs for breakfast, a whole avocado for lunch, and an apple for a snack (see chapter 6 for menu planning and recipes). Food doesn't have to be complicated or difficult. Instead of making an elaborate meal, eat a fresh salad, which costs less and is better for you than processed, sugar-laden products.

Farmer's markets are great venues to find fresh, local produce. It is best to eat locally grown fruit and vegetables whenever possible. Buy a potato and bake it with the following toppings: olive oil, broccoli, scallions, and sea salt with kelp. The baked potato is better for you than a bag of potato chips. Eat foods closer to their original harvested form.

Food Labeling

When you start this gluten-free journey, learn to read food labels to ensure you do not ingest gluten. You become a detective perusing each label to find hidden sources, since gluten is labeled using many names (see the list below). Unfortunately, manufacturers can randomly change ingredients, so make it a practice to read labels each time you shop.

Since derivatives of wheat, rye, and barley go by numerous names, it makes the GF transition harder (see the Questionable Foods section in this chapter). The label may identify them as additives, flavorings, or seasonings. In medications they may be called fillers or binders and could be in both over-the-counter and prescription meds (see the Medications section in this chapter). So grab the magnifying glass, Sherlock Holmes, and read that label.

Since manufacturers caught onto the GF trend, many now label their gluten-free items. If a food is not labeled GF, check the ingredients. Look for the following gluten-containing ingredients on each food label:

- Barley
- Dextrin
- Dinkle
- Durum
- Emmer
- Farro
- Farina
- Malt
- Natural flavoring
- Oats (unless labeled gluten-free)
- Rye
- Spelt
- Triticale
- Wheat

One ingredient that sounds like it might contain gluten is maltodextrin. However, it does not because it is made from corn.

Cross-contamination may occur in grocery store bulk bins. Bin scoops used for a gluten-containing product may be used by a customer for a GF item. Consequently, you should avoid purchasing items from bulk bins.

It may be helpful to download a gluten-free shopping guide app on your phone. Some apps contain an extensive list of GF items from grocery stores as well as restaurants. Also, celiac.com contains lists of safe and gluten-containing foods. Any assistance with understanding the label detective work is helpful.

Top Food Allergens

Food companies are required by law to list highly allergic foods on their labels, including wheat. Unfortunately, this does not include gluten. The Food Allergen Labeling and Consumer Protection Act (FALCPA) requires food manufacturers to list these eight most common food allergens:

- Eggs
- Fish
- Milk
- Nuts
- Peanuts
- Shellfish
- Soy
- Wheat

Therefore, if a product contains one of these ingredients, it must be listed on the label. The manufacturer can include an allergy statement after the list of ingredients that usually begins with the word *contains*.

Or the allergen can be listed in the ingredient list, requiring you to read the label. Any food containing wheat should be clearly labeled.

Food and Drug Administration

The Food and Drug Administration's (FDA) gluten-free labeling regulations apply to dairy products and canned, frozen, and packaged foods. According to the FDA, manufacturers should test GF products to ensure they contain less than 20 parts per million (ppm) of gluten, which could still cause problems for some people. Manufacturers can be fined for not complying with this standard. Foods labeled GF also guarantee against cross-contamination at the manufacturing facility.

Why can't prepackaged GF foods be completely void of gluten? It would be almost impossible for food manufacturers to ensure this because they may not grow the produce or transport it to their facility. Therefore, cross-contamination could occur outside of the factory. Twenty ppm is the lowest amount that can be reliably detected in foods. This is why the only guaranteed GF foods are whole naturally GF foods.

Manufacturers are not required to label foods that may be exposed to cross-contamination. However, some voluntarily include warnings such as "manufactured in a factory that also processes wheat." If this is on the label, do not purchase it. Unfortunately, you won't see warnings about cross-contamination for oats, barley, or rye because they are not one of the top eight food allergens.

Gluten-free labeling has come a long way. It is easier to figure out whether an item contains wheat or gluten now than it did a decade ago. As you peruse the grocery aisles, notice how many food labels include gluten-free on the package.

United States Department of Agriculture

The United States Department of Agriculture (USDA) governs food regulation for meat, poultry, and eggs. The USDA does not make it mandatory for manufacturers to list allergens on the label.

However, it is encouraged. Raw, unprocessed eggs and meat do not naturally contain gluten, but gluten-containing ingredients can be added to them. For example, marinated meats from the grocery store most likely contain gluten.

Alcohol and Tobacco Tax and Trade Bureau

The Alcohol and Tobacco Tax and Trade Bureau (TTB) regulates the labeling of alcoholic beverages. The TTB encourages manufacturers to list allergens such as wheat, but it is not required. The TTB only allows gluten-free labeling on alcoholic beverages that also meet the FDA definition of gluten-free—the 20 ppm and made from ingredients that don't contain gluten.

Foods to Eliminate

Understanding what foods contain gluten is crucial if you have a gluten-related disorder. Since foods may contain hidden sources of gluten, you should investigate labels and search the Internet to find out whether a food contains gluten. For example, Ginny began experiencing digestive issues while taking Tylenol, and when she researched it, she discovered that it contains gluten. Now she purchases a generic brand of acetaminophen that is GF. As you begin your transition to a GF diet, begin to eliminate the following foods that contain gluten.

Alcoholic Beverages

Wine is made from grapes, so it is GF. However, wine coolers, ciders, sangria, and other beverages containing wine could have gluten ingredients added to them. Beers, ales, lagers, and malt beverages contain gluten. However, some breweries produce GF options.

Supposedly, all distilled liquors such as brandy, bourbon, cognac, gin, rum, schnapps, tequila, vodka, and whiskey are GF because the distillation process removes the gluten. However, some of these alcohols are made from wheat, barley, or rye. The TTB does not allow gluten-free labeling on beverages made from these ingredients. Ginny drinks only verified GF alcohol such as Deep Eddies and Tito's vodka as well as 100 percent agave tequila. Also, Chopin vodka is made from potatoes, and Ciroc vodka is made from grapes. Flavored liquors usually contain gluten.

Baked Goods

Most baked goods such as cakes, cobblers, cookies, bagels, biscuits, brownies, muffins, donuts, crackers, piecrust, and pastries contain gluten. It is possible to bake your own GF versions. Check out recipes on the Satisfying Eats Blog at SatisfyingEats.com.

Barley

Barley is a grain commonly used in bread, soups, stews, and alcoholic beverages. Pearled barley is similar to the texture of brown rice.

Beer

Unless is it labeled GF, beer contains gluten.

Bread

Any bread made from wheat, barley, or rye, such as bagels, croissants, cornbread, donuts, flatbreads, muffins, pita, pizza crust, and rolls, contains gluten.

Breading and Coating Mixes

Most breading and coating mixes are made from wheat.

. . .

Breakfast Foods

Bagels, biscuits, crepes, French toast, pancakes, toast, and waffles are most likely made from wheat. Omelets at restaurants may contain gluten (see omelets below).

Brown Rice Syrup

This ingredient may be made with barley.

Candy and Candy Bars

Many forms of candy include malt, malt flavoring, malt extract, wheat flour, or wheat starch, which contain gluten. Chocolate usually contains gluten. Check the label for the ingredient malt (see malt below).

Cereal

Many types of cereals have gluten. Read the label. Gluten-free cereals usually contain 20 ppm of gluten, so do not eat too much in one day.

Chapstick

Check the label to see if it contains a hidden source of gluten. When you use lip products, you can ingest small amounts of it when eating or drinking. Ingesting gluten through these products can cause symptoms.

Cheesecake

Some recipes contain wheat.

Chips

Most chips do not contain gluten unless they are flavored. Check the label's ingredients.

Coffee

Coffee is naturally gluten-free. However, flavored coffee, coffee drinks, and flavored creamers may contain gluten.

Communion Wafers

Most communion wafers are made from wheat flour. However, many religious establishments provide a GF substitute.

Cookie Dough

Cookie dough usually contains wheat. It may be included in ice cream or premade to be cooked at home.

Crackers

Graham crackers, saltine crackers, goldfish, pretzels, and most other crackers contain wheat. Stores carry gluten-free pretzels and crackers.

Couscous

This type of grain is derived from wheat.

Cream of Wheat

Of course this hot breakfast cereal contains wheat.

Croutons

Croutons are usually made from bread.

. . .

Dairy Substitutes

Some types of dairy substitutes contain gluten. Read the label.

Energy Bars/Granola Bars

Many granola or protein bars contain some form of gluten. Check the label. GF varieties are available, but don't overeat in one day, as it may contain 20 ppm of gluten.

Flour

Most flour is made from wheat. However, you can find many GF options such as coconut and almond flour.

French Fries

Even though potatoes do not contain gluten, the fryer may be used for items that do contain gluten (a batter), so there would be cross-contamination. However, some restaurants have GF fryers, so ask.

Granola

Most granola products are made with regular oats versus GF oats. Regular oats may contain gluten due to cross-contamination. If you buy the GF variety, it may contain 20 ppm per serving. Limit your number of servings. Granola may also contain malt (see malt).

Groats

Check to see if the groats are made from wheat, barley, rye, or oats (that are not GF).

. . .

Gravy

Most gravies, sauces, and roux contain gluten.

Gum

You can't be sure that gum does not contain gluten unless it is labeled gluten-free.

Flavored Foods

Many flavored foods contain gluten due to the flavoring, such as coffee, chips, syrups, whipped toppings, coffee creamers, and sprinkles.

Imitation Crab Meat

Gluten binds it together.

Lipstick, Lip Gloss, Lip Balm

Similar to chapstick, these products could contain a hidden source of gluten and cause symptoms.

Lunch Meat

Most forms of lunch meat include gluten unless it specifically states GF.

Malt

Malt is made from a grain (barley, wheat, corn, rice) that has been soaked, sprouted, and dried. Since barley is the most common grain used, beware of foods containing malt. Malt comes in various forms such as:

- Brewer's malt
- Malt extract
- Malt flavoring
- Malted milkshake
- Malt syrup
- Malt vinegar

Many chocolates, cereals, granolas, beverages, baked goods, and herbal teas contain malt.

Marinades

Marinades and teriyaki contain gluten.

Meats

Preseasoned meats and poultry that have been injected or self-basted may contain gluten. Sausage may contain seasonings that contain gluten. Chicken and turkey might contain gluten if injected with a plumping solution. Make sure chicken is not molded into a premade, unnatural patty, which contains gluten.

Meat Substitutes

Vegetarian burgers, sausage, and imitation bacon or seafood usually contain gluten.

Medications

Prescriptions, over the counter medications, and supplements may contain wheat starch. The starch helps to bind the ingredients in the pill. Unfortunately, there are no labeling requirements regarding gluten for medications. Therefore, search the Internet to determine whether the item contains gluten. A brand medication may contain gluten, whereas the generic version does not or vice versa. Tell your pharmacist that you are GF when filling prescription drugs.

Millet

This grain is naturally gluten-free. However, it may be processed in the same plant as wheat so it could become cross-contaminated. Purchase millet that is GF.

Noodles

Most varieties of noodles are made from wheat, including egg noodles, ramen, soba, spaghetti, and udon. Grocery stores carry an abundant variety of GF noodles.

Oats

Oats are naturally gluten-free. However, cross-contamination may occur if processed in the same plant or shipped in the same vehicle as wheat. Some individuals with celiac disease elicit a similar immune response to the protein in oats as in gluten. If you use oats make sure they are certified gluten-free because they are grown, harvested, and processed with dedicated GF machinery.

Oil

Make sure the oil you purchase does not contain gluten because some flavored oils do.

Omelets at Restaurants

Some restaurants use an omelet mix that may contain gluten, or they may add pancake mix to the omelet to make it fluffy. Ask the restaurant staff.

. . .

Pancakes and Waffles

These breakfast foods are usually made from wheat flour. However, you can make these items at home with GF flour. Gluten-free pancake and muffin mixes are available but may contain up to 20 ppm, so don't overindulge.

Pasta

Most pasta such as spaghetti, ravioli, tortellini, gnocchi, orzo, and dumplings are made from wheat. Supermarkets do carry many GF varieties derived from other foods.

Peanut Butter

Check the label and ensure it does not contain gluten additives. It should be labeled gluten-free.

Play-Doh®

This item may not be in your pantry, but you need to know that it contains gluten. Martin (Introduction story) kept having gluten-related symptoms when his grandchildren would visit. Finally, he figured out it was due to the Play-Doh® he took out for them to use. He got rid of the Play-Doh®. Find a gluten-free play-dough recipe on the Internet if you want to make it for the kids in your life.

Potato Chips

Seasoned potato chips may contain malt vinegar or wheat starch—hidden sources of gluten.

Rye

The gluten-containing grain rye is used to make rye bread, crackers, and whiskey.

Salad Dressings

Gluten is used to thicken salad dressings. Read the label to verify whether your dressing is GF. Instead, use oil and vinegar, especially at restaurants.

Sauces

Gluten is used as a thickening agent for most sauces. Be suspicious of any sauce.

Soups

Soups and broths may be thickened with gluten too.

Soy Sauce

Soy sauce contains gluten. Stores carry GF options. Tamari made without wheat is GF. Coconut amino is a GF replacement for soy sauce.

Spice Blends

In spice blends, gluten prevents the ingredients from clumping together. Most spices have GF versions. Question every spice put on your food, especially when eating out.

Stuffing

Stuffing and dressing are primarily made from wheat.

. . .

Sushi

Sushi may or may not contain gluten. Ask if soy sauce was used when preparing it. Make sure any vinegar used to prepare the rice was GF (see vinegar).

Tabbouleh

This delicious Middle Eastern salad is made with bulgur wheat.

Tamari

Tamari contains gluten unless it is labeled as GF.

Tea

Many herbal teas contain malt. Check the label.

Teriyaki Sauce

Teriyaki is made with soy sauce, which usually contains gluten unless labeled GF.

Toothpaste

Numerous manufacturers make GF toothpaste, but not all kinds of toothpastes are GF. Read the label or search the Internet to find a brand that is GF.

Tortillas

Tortillas made from wheat contain gluten. However, GF options are available. If you choose to buy corn tortillas, make sure they do not contain gluten.

. . .

Wheat

Thousands of products in the grocery store contain wheat. Foods with breadings and coatings are usually made from it.

There are different varieties of wheat so you should become familiar with their names:

- Duram or durum
- Einkorn
- Emmer
- Farina
- Farro
- Kamut
- Semolina
- Spelt
- Triticum

Wheat can also be processed and go by these names:

- Bulgar or bulgur wheat
- Disodium wheatgermamido Peg-2 sulfosuccinate
- Graham flour
- Hydrolyzed wheat protein
- Kibbled wheat
- Matzoh, matzah, and matzo
- Seitan or kofu
- Vital wheat gluten
- Wheat berries
- Wheat bran
- Wheat germ
- Wheat protein
- Wheat starch

Vinegar

White, red, balsamic, and apple cider vinegar do not contain gluten. However, some rice vinegars from Asia may contain a mixture of grains. Vinegar made only from rice is GF. Seasoned or blended vinegars (include more than one source) often contain added flavors that may not be GF. Malt vinegar contains gluten.

Yeast

Brewer's yeast contains gluten. However, the yeast used for bread or nutritional yeast does not.

Questionable Foods

Since the FDA requires manufacturers to label wheat, you can be sure wheat byproducts are labeled. However, derivatives of rye, barley, and oats (may be cross-contaminated) can be labeled by many names. The alias names make it difficult to identify if the product contains gluten or not. Therefore, the following list of ingredients is questionable:

- Enzymes
- Fillers
- Flavors
- Natural flavors
- Modified food starch
- Rice malt (if made from barley)
- Seasonings
- Spices
- Stabilizers
- Starch
- Wheatgrass (if it contains seeds, it has gluten)

These ingredients listed above may or may not contain gluten. Manufacturers can label barley malt as flavors or natural flavoring. Therefore, if a food contains one of these questionable ingredients, use your app, resources, or the Internet to find out whether the product contains gluten. If you cannot find the answer, do not purchase it.

At first your grocery shopping trips may be time-consuming. However, in no time you will get the hang of checking labels. The following label checking tips may help:

1. Check for gluten-free on the front.
2. Read the ingredient list to see if it says "contains wheat."
3. Scan the ingredient list for wheat (or one of the other wheat names listed above).
4. Check for barley, oats, rye, malt, or soy.
5. If the label includes a name from the questionable list, investigate further.

Reading processed food labels is challenging since it's hard to pronounce many of the multisyllable words. However, after reading the chemicals contained in processed foods, maybe you won't want to buy them.

Label reading is much easier than it used to be because of the regulations and labeling of GF products. Manufacturers have caught on and add labels to products even if they are naturally gluten-free. Before you know it, you will become a label scanning pro.

Clean Out the Kitchen

Now it is time to transition to a GF kitchen. Gluten-free food mustn't come into contact with a surface in your kitchen that has a gluten residue. Therefore, it is essential to clean and organize the kitchen.

You should remove or separate everything that contains gluten for two reasons—cross-contamination and temptation. Packages of cookies or other sweet treats can cause someone to indulge in foods containing gluten. Just looking at the bag releases dopamine and an overwhelming desire to consume that food.[1] Therefore, it is best to remove these items from your home or place them out of sight. If a family member wants to eat foods that tempt you, they should keep these packages hidden in their room or on a shelf high in the pantry. Ask them to honor your goals and help you in this way.

Sorting through food in the kitchen is not the tough part of this process. It's the cleaning that can be overwhelming. Think of gluten as a glue. If a gluten-containing item touched anything in your kitchen, it leaves a sticky gluten residue. Therefore, all items must be scrubbed or thrown away if the invisible gluten grime cannot be removed. If this initial cleaning does not occur, you may continue to ingest small amounts of gluten.

Unfortunately, the dishwasher is not strong enough to remove the sticky gluten. You have to scrub the surface of each item that has had contact with gluten-containing foods. So fill that sink full of sudsy water and start scrubbing.

Ginny continued to experience digestive symptoms until she thoroughly completed the kitchen cleaning process. This process was one of her missing puzzle pieces. She figured out that gluten stuck to plastic kitchen items such as measuring cups, colanders, and plastic storage containers. Therefore, she threw away her plastic dishes and utensils and replaced them with metal, glass, ceramic, and other nonporous kitchen gadgets.

The cleaning process can be daunting for one person. Therefore, I suggest you solicit help from a family member or friend, or hire someone. If you have support, that person can clean while you sort through food, and you'll complete the job in half the time. As you assess kitchen gadgets, toss stuff you do not use. Your cabinets will shine, and it will seem like you have a new kitchen. As a reward for your hard work—your symptoms will subside. Your effort is well worth the relief you will attain.

Clean Out Cross-Contamination Items and Areas

Your kitchen contains many places and items that contain residue from gluten. This list will help you identify the sources so you can clean, replace, or replicate the item. For example, you may want to own a GF toaster. For the following items, purchase new ones for GF foods only:

- Bread machine
- Can opener
- Colanders
- Containers
- Cutting boards
- Fryers
- Measuring cups, spoons (replace if plastic)
- Pots/pans/baking pans/muffin tins (replace if nonstick)
- Rolling pin (replace if wooden)
- Salad tongs (replace if wooden or plastic)
- Sifters
- Sippy cups
- Skillets (replace if nonstick or cast iron)
- Spatula (replace if nylon, plastic, or silicon)
- Stone bakeware
- Strainer
- Toaster
- Toaster oven
- Waffle iron
- Wooden utensils

You only need to replace the item if it will be used for preparing gluten-free foods. A scratched nonstick pot or pan could harbor gluten. Purchase new pots that do not have a nonstick surface. Rounded corner baking dishes are easier to clean. Label the new items for GF use only with a permanent marker. It may be helpful to store these objects in a GF cabinet to avoid cross-contamination.

Pretend the gluten grime is all over the kitchen. If you ever baked with flour, it is everywhere since flour can be airborne. All the surfaces in your kitchen need to be sanitized.

Take everything out of each kitchen cabinet and scrub or toss it. Wipe the cabinet surfaces—including the bottom, sides, and top of each shelf—with a dishwashing liquid and warm-water solution. All the items from inside the cabinet need to be scrubbed or wiped down before putting them back. Your kitchen will be as clean as when you moved in.

When washing baking pans, be sure to scrub the corners where dried baked goods can lodge. Carefully clean the seams around pan lids. Clean countertops, utensil drawers, and refrigerator shelves often to remove crumbs. Wash sponges and dishtowels after they come into contact with gluten.

Clean Out the Pantry

Now that you cleaned your kitchen and all the cabinets, it is time to tackle the pantry. First, take everything out of one shelf of the pantry and thoroughly clean it like you did the cabinets. Next, using the list of gluten-containing foods recorded earlier in this chapter, read the label of each pantry item to determine if it contains gluten. If it does, you may choose to throw it out, give it away, or place it on a gluten-designated shelf in the pantry. Before you put it back, be sure to wipe it to remove the gluten grime thoroughly.

You may want to place tempting gluten-containing snacks on a high pantry shelf out of sight. However, place wheat flours on a lower shelf so the wheat residue does not float down onto GF foods when you remove it from the shelf. Keep wheat flour in a ziplock bag to decrease cross-contamination.

In addition to sorting through gluten items from your pantry, you may want to evaluate the refined carbohydrate and sugar level of your foods before you put them back. If you want to improve your health by decreasing your sugar and processed food consumption, remove the following items:

- Sugar-sweetened drinks—like soda, fruit juice, Gatorade (Flavored waters with no calories are okay to keep and finish, but after they are gone it is best to drink water. If you need to, add a slice of lemon and stevia to your water.)
- Sugar—white sugar, high-fructose corn syrup—remove any item with greater than 10 grams of sugar per serving. Unfortunately, sugar does not have a recommended daily allowance.
- Rice—white rice (brown and wild rice are fine)
- Corn—all non-organic corn products such as tortilla chips and popcorn (Organic corn products are fine to consume.)
- Artificial sweeteners—saccharin, aspartame or Equal/NutraSweet, sucralose or Splenda (It is okay to keep honey, maple syrup, agave, stevia, xylitol, coconut sugar, and monk fruit sugar.)
- Oils—eliminate all oils except olive oil (use when cooking at low temperatures) and coconut oil (use when cooking at high temperatures)
- Any processed food in a box or bag—such as chips, crackers, cookies, and cereal, unless it is organic and you choose to make this an exception
- Foods containing partially hydrogenated vegetable oil, high-fructose corn syrup, or monosodium glutamate (MSG). Food labels disguise MSG through the following names: flavors; flavoring; enzymes; hydrolyzed, autolyzed

yeast; barley malt; hydrolyzed vegetable protein; maltodextrin; natural seasonings; and glutamate.

Clean Out the Refrigerator and Freezer

Let's move on to cleaning out the refrigerator. Again, remove all the items from one shelf in your fridge and freezer at a time, going through the same process as the pantry. If you choose to keep any gluten-containing foods, put them on a separate shelf. Wipe each item off before returning it to the fridge.

Old condiments may be contaminated because a utensil used on a gluten-containing food may have been redipped into a condiment. Purchase new gluten-free condiments designated for the GF individual, and label them. You could use a permanent marker or label maker.

If you want to improve your health and weight remove the following unhealthy items from your refrigerator to decrease your sugar and refined carbohydrate consumption:

.

- Wheat products
- Processed meats such as ham, bacon, sausage, hot dogs, and lunch meat
- Soft drinks and fruit juices—they are loaded with sugar
- Check the ingredients of condiments. If one contains high-fructose corn syrup, throw it out. Health-food stores carry better condiment substitutes, such as organic mayonnaise.
- Margarine—organic butter is a healthier choice
- All milk products except plain Greek yogurt, which contains probiotics
- Packaged frozen meals (while convenient, even "healthy" brands of frozen foods are processed)

From this point on, cleanliness is fundamental, so be diligent to wipe off surfaces, pantry shelves, and refrigerator shelves and scrub dishes that come into contact with gluten.

Clean Out the Medicine Cabinet

Since supplements, over-the-counter medications, and prescription drugs can contain gluten, you need to clean out this area too. Again, take everything out of the cabinet, wipe it down, and read every label. Use a permanent marker to write "GF" or "contains gluten." Clean and organize the area now, versus when you are sick.

Clean Out Your Emotions

Food and emotions are intrinsically tied together for most of us, so we need to do an emotional check when we begin to clean out the gluten provisions that have previously brought us comfort. Food can be used for the wrong reasons. We may eat because we are sad, bored, stressed out, depressed, or happy. As we engage in emotional eating, we turn to food to appease ourselves. If we feel abandoned, food can be our friend. We can swallow our angry feelings with food, instead of feeling the emotions we don't want to deal with. Food can provide an emotional escape from negative feelings.

To help you gain more awareness regarding emotional eating, document why you eat. Is it because of hunger or to relieve stress? Record any negative emotions you experience and determine if you eat because of your feelings. Do you have a deep emotional wound that needs healing? Is there someone you need to forgive? Maybe you have a big hole in your heart that you are filling with food. Connect the dots between your eating habits and emotions. If you need additional help, feel free to join my private Facebook group: 7 Steps to Get Off Sugar and Carbohydrates (https://www.facebook.com/groups/184355458927013/about/). I am also a certified health and wellness coach and provide services through my website at http://christianyoga.com/coaching.

Sometimes we engage in mindless eating and munch on something without being hungry. When bored, we may look in the refrigerator or pantry but can't find anything appealing. If this happens to you, food is not what you need. First, drink two glasses of water, as you may be thirsty and don't realize it.

Are you eating because of a negative emotion you do not want to deal with? If you are an emotional eater, don't escape from negative feelings through food. Instead, recognize dysfunctional eating behaviors and confront tough issues in your life. Each time you recognize emotional eating, clean out your emotions. Then you can disengage the connection between eating and feelings.

Stress also causes us to turn to food. We live in a fast-paced world where we eat on the run. We no longer have traditional meals prepared from scratch at home. Unfortunately, we are letting food industries cook our food for us. What is causing you stress? What can you change or eliminate to reduce stress in your life?

Becoming aware of emotional or stress eating is half the battle. When you recognize you are about to emotionally eat or eat out of stress, set the timer for ten minutes and do something to distract yourself. Go for a walk, call a friend, turn on the TV, or drink a glass of water. Develop strategies to use when you need to distract yourself from eating. Plan ahead to avoid emotional and stress eating. Prepare your weekly menu (see chapter 6), and have healthy snacks on hand so you do not grab that convenient gluten-filled one.

Summary

Try not to be overwhelmed by the amount of information or work you need to do to begin and maintain a GF lifestyle. You can get this done little by little. A couple of months from now, reading labels will be second nature. Your spotless kitchen will seem brand-new again. As you eat a GF diet, your symptoms will be relieved. Walk confidently toward this healthier lifestyle.

Make sure you take the following action steps. Schedule a date to clean out your kitchen, pantry, refrigerator, freezer, and medicine cabinet.

Date to clean out:

Kitchen _____

Pantry _____

Refrigerator _____

Freezer _____

Medicine Cabinet_____

The next chapter, Menu Planning and Recipes, will guide you to the foods you need to purchase and teach you to plan menus to implement this new lifestyle. You are embarking on one of the best lifestyle changes. Embrace the GF way of living.

6

MENU PLANNING AND RECIPES

Michael's Story

Michael was a healthy, breastfed eight-month-old boy until he began eating solid foods. His mother introduced rice cereal first, as the pediatrician suggested. After a month, Michael started eating wheat cereal. A few weeks later, he got his first ear infection and became fussy. His doctor treated the infection with amoxicillin.

His parents thought their child's irritability was due to teething. Holding and rocking did not appease his poor temperament. A month later, he developed a second ear infection and was prescribed a second antibiotic. His stools loosened and lost form, leading his parents to believe these symptoms were due to the antibiotics. He cried constantly and wanted to be held all the time.

Michael's immune system was so compromised he contracted respiratory syncytial virus (RSV). He ran fevers with profuse nasal congestion and was sick and inconsolable for weeks. Eventually, his illness progressed to pneumonia and subsequent hospitalization, where he received intravenous fluids and antibiotics.

At his twelve-month pediatrician visit, Michael's weight had dropped from the 50 percentile on the growth chart down to the 5 percentile. He continued to suffer from diarrhea. The doctor suspected celiac disease since the child's array of symptoms started the month wheat was introduced into *his diet. However, the results of a gluten antibody blood test were negative. The pediatrician still suspected celiac disease, so Michael had an upper GI diagnostic test under general anesthesia. But the biopsies from his small intestine showed his villi were normal. The doctor then suspected failure to thrive, yet during Michael's first eight months he was never sick, of average weight, and generally happy and content.*

By eighteen months Michael's temperament had also changed dramatically from what it was at eight months. His parents thought he might be autistic. When he wasn't crying, he stared into space and appeared lethargic. Michael stopped interacting, was persistently cranky, and suffered from continued diarrhea. He saw the doctor often for reoccurring ear infections and was prescribed course after course of antibiotics.

When Michael was twenty months old, a friend of his parents suggested they try a gluten-free diet in case he was gluten-sensitive, in spite of the lack of a definitive celiac diagnosis. After only three days of eating GF, Michael quit crying, and his temperament improved. After a week, his loose bowel movements stopped, and his stools gained form. A few weeks later, he began interacting normally again. Michael was diagnosed with non-celiac gluten sensitivity.

In chapter 5 you learned how to embrace the gluten-free diet through cleaning and preparing your kitchen. All the knowledge you gained regarding what foods contain gluten will be used in this chapter as you plan your menu and prepare to grocery shop.

You do not have to deprive yourself when eating a GF diet. Lobster, filet mignon, and salmon paired with brussels sprouts, asparagus, or broccoli are not depriving. When transitioning to eating GF, it is best to start with foods that are naturally GF. Therefore, this chapter provides many options for you to create delicious GF meals.

Preparing and eating meals at home is best when transitioning to a new way of eating. You know exactly what is going into every dish, including seasonings. You do not need advanced skills to cook GF—merely a recipe and the ingredients. I've included fifty GF recipes in appendix 3. Since you cleaned your kitchen, you should not run into cross-contamination with gluten-containing foods like you might when eating out. Chapter 7 will guide you with dining at restaurants.

If you have a gluten-related disorder, you may also be lactose intolerant. If the lining of your small intestine is inflamed, it may not produce enough lactose, which is a natural sugar in milk. Without this enzyme you can't properly digest milk products. Instead you experience gas, bloating, abdominal pain, and diarrhea. Fortunately, after you stop eating gluten, your small intestine heals, and for some people lactose intolerance resolves. Initially, when you begin eating a GF diet, you should also stop consuming milk products; this will allow your gastrointestinal tract to heal. It took a while for Michaels's GI tract to heal.

Healthy Foods to Purchase

When planning your menu, choose a rich selection of healthy foods. Focus on eating groceries that are naturally gluten-free—fresh vegetables, fruits, beans, GF grains, nuts, seeds, meats, and eggs. Each food group provides essential nutrients the body needs to function at its highest potential.

There are over a hundred different vegetables because the human body needs various types of nutrients for proper growth and performance. For example, spinach contains vitamins A and K, whereas broccoli is full of vitamin E. Choose variety to ensure you get the appropriate amounts of fiber, vitamins, and minerals.

Grains provide carbohydrates the body uses for fuel or energy, similar to gas in a car. An assortment of GF grains includes amaranth, buckwheat, millet, quinoa, brown rice, teff, and wild rice. I do not recommend white rice because of the way it is processed today, with the nutrients stripped away; all others are beneficial and naturally GF.

Nuts are excellent sources of protein, similar to meat. Choose from the following varieties—almond, brazil, cashew, chestnut, hazelnut, macadamia, pecan, pistachio, pine, and walnut. Be sure to buy raw nuts because they contain more nutrition in their natural GF form, instead of roasted, salted, or sugar-coated, which could contain gluten. Instead, taste the natural flavor of almonds, pecans, and walnuts. Nuts are full of omega-3 oils, which are essential for brain function.

Peanuts are not a nut but a type of vegetable called a legume (i.e., pea or bean). They grow in the ground and don't come from a tree. I do not recommend consuming products made with peanuts because they are hard to digest, and many people are allergic to them. Other legumes (beans, lentils, and peas) may be difficult for some people to digest, but generally don't cause allergic reactions.

Seeds are full of trace minerals the human body needs but in small amounts. Chia, flax, hemp, poppy, pumpkin, sesame, and sunflower seeds are all naturally GF.

Fruits are sweet and delicious and provide the body with the fiber, vitamins, and minerals our bodies need to be healthy. Instead of eating a dish of ice cream, eat a juicy strawberry, tangy green apple, or crunchy pomegranate.

Fruits and vegetables are seasonal, which means each season (spring, summer, fall, winter) different crops are harvested. In the south, strawberries ripen in early spring. Okra and peas grow best in the summer. Pumpkins mature in the fall. Citrus fruit is picked in the winter when our bodies require more vitamin C to prevent colds. We should eat the ones that ripen in that season. Not only will we get the nutrients we need for that season but we won't tire of the same type of foods all year long.

Sometimes we get into the habit of eating similar foods over and over again, but it is healthier to eat an assortment to take in a variety of nutrients. We can choose from a vast number of vegetables, grains, nuts, seeds, and fruits that are naturally GF and unique in their flavors and amounts of nutrients. These options not only provide what our body needs but they are delicious to enjoy as well.

Processed foods from boxes or bags may have been sitting on the shelves for months, and many contain gluten, which is used to bind the ingredients together. Instead, we need a vast selection of fresh food since our bodies need a broad range of nutrients to function correctly. By eating different foods from each food category (vegetable, fruit, grain, nut, seed), you take proper care of your body.

When you purchase meat, make sure it is organic, grass fed, or free range with no hormones or antibiotics. Do not buy meats that are coated with a marinade, breaded, or seasoned, as they may contain gluten. Antibiotics we consume from meat may harm our gut flora.

We do not need to consume meat at every meal. Too much protein in a person's diet causes the body to extract calcium from the bones and send it into the bloodstream to balance its pH.[1] This calcium leaching weakens a person's bones and is a factor in osteoporosis. In fact, incidences of osteoporosis in third-world countries with a low-protein diet are lower than industrialized nations.[2]

One summer I bought a new fruit and vegetable every week at the grocery store. It was an excellent experience for my children and me as I got out of the rut of cooking the same meals over and over, and we discovered different foods we liked such as red cabbage, star fruit, and bok choy.

Menu Planning

Weekly planning is essential to successfully implement the GF lifestyle. Choose a quiet spot to plan your menu and corresponding grocery list. This may take up to an hour. I usually do this on Sunday afternoons. If the weather is nice, I sit by the pool and get my vitamin D naturally from the sun. Use this book, another healthy GF cookbook, or an app on your phone to find recipes. I recommend the *Comforting Eats* cookbook (grain-free, sugar-free, and hunger-free recipes) by Melissa Monroe McGehee at SatisfyingEats.com. To get you started, I've listed fifty GF recipes in appendix 3.

When cooking, most recipes can be adapted to eliminate gluten.

Instead of thickening your grandmother's soup recipe with flour, use cornstarch or arrowroot powder, which are naturally GF. The GF version of the recipe can be just as delicious. For example, a recipe that calls for a breadcrumb coating can be prepared with crushed nuts instead. The nut version may taste better and have a higher nutritional value. If you like baked goods, the *Satisfying Eats* cookbook perfected them, and it contains over sixty dessert recipes that are low in sugar and GF.

When you bake without gluten you need to have just the right amount of ingredients so the item does not crumble and is not too dense. Finding a great GF cookbook solves this problem. Creating a large batch of a GF flour mixture is smart. It saves you time when you want to make pancakes or waffles. If you make your own, you know what it is in it.

If you purchase the premade GF flours in the stores, many will contain up to the 20 ppm of gluten per serving. However, a premade, store-bought flour may be most convenient for you at this time. Avoid using mixes containing white rice flour and potato starch flour since manufacturers strip the nutrients from these products, and they are high in refined carbohydrates. Healthy GF flours include those made from almonds, coconuts, quinoa, amaranth, brown rice, teff, garbanzo beans, sorghum, or buckwheat. These flours contain the whole grain and are not processed like white rice. The grain buckwheat does not contain wheat or gluten, despite its name.

Become creative with vegetables as a bread substitute. For example, romaine lettuce could be the shell for your tacos. The taco fixings fit inside the boat shape of the lettuce well. You could add GF barbeque beef to a baked potato instead of a bun. Red cabbage leaves are great for sandwiches. Appendix 3 includes a recipe for sandwiches that use blanched collard green leaves as the wrap. What other foods could be used as a bread substitute? Get creative.

Each week I list what I plan to cook for breakfast, lunch, dinner, and snack for every day of the week. As I choose a recipe, I write down the corresponding ingredients I need on my grocery list. For years, as my children were growing up, I posted on their chalkboard the menu for every day of the week. Everyone in the family knew what I would be serving. I cooked on Sunday and Monday and listed leftovers (from Sunday) to be served on Tuesday. Wednesday we all ate at church, and Thursday I served leftovers from Monday. Two nights of cooking took care of four meals. To liven up leftovers, I cooked one new item (such as a vegetable) to go along with the previous meal and to add new interest.

I created a standard grocery list for the store I used. To create this list, initially I walked through the store and either wrote or dictated into my phone notes the aisles and the items I normally purchased on each aisle. For example, I would start in the back of the store in the refrigerated section and include eggs, butter, coconut milk, kefir, and Greek yogurt on the list for that aisle. Then I proceeded to the next aisle, cleaning supplies and paper products. I listed Clorox wipes, toilet paper, napkins, paper towels, paper plates, etc. And so on, until I had a master grocery list compiled. At home, I typed out this list based on each grocery store aisle and the products I normally purchased. It took work to create this list, but it has streamlined my grocery store planning for years.

Today you will find a vast array of gluten-free choices compared to a decade ago. Some stores even have a dedicated GF section. If you can't find something at the grocery store, order it online. Check out the online store Gluten-Free Mall at https://www.glutenfreemall.com/catalog/.

Each week I printed a fresh new grocery list, and my family knew that if we ran out of an item, they circled it on the list or wrote it out. I made a rule to guide us in shopping: if it wasn't on the list, it didn't get purchased. That put some responsibility on them, not all on me.

Every week I made a large, fresh, raw salad (broccoli salad, beet salad, cole slaw, salad with lettuce) and I ate that for lunch each day. For my children's lunch boxes, I tried to include one fresh fruit and vegetable. When they wanted a fruit roll-up, I explained that they had something better in a real piece of fruit (their choice) because it was loaded with natural vitamins and minerals to nourish their bodies. My children learned the importance of whole foods.

Post your menu on the refrigerator so you know what you planned to cook for each meal during the week. Next, hit the grocery store or local farmer's market. Your family will appreciate your planning and food preparation, and being prepared will keep you from making unhealthy impulsive choices when you grocery shop. After you purchase all those groceries, it is time to start cooking healthy home-made gluten-free meals.

Meal Planning

To assist you with this transition, GF meal ideas are listed below. Appendix 3 contains corresponding recipes. The following meal categories are healthy and GF. These options will help you create your menu and shopping list.

Breakfast

- Avocado Egg Bake
- Bacon, Lettuce, Scrambled Eggs
- Bacon-Wrapped Green Apples
- Berry Smoothie
- Eggs Benedict
- Mushroom Frittata
- Omelet
- Prosciutto Wrapped Pears
- Spinach Topped Eggs
- Poultry Patties
- Hard-boiled eggs

Breakfast Breads

- Apple Quinoa Breakfast Muffins
- Blueberry-Lemon Muffins
- Cinnamon Bread
- Strawberry/Almond Coffee Cake

Lunch

- Apple Coleslaw
- Bison Burgers
- Chicken Collard Wraps
- Deviled Eggs
- Kale Butternut Salad
- Quinoa Salad
- Sweet Potato Spinach Salad
- Salad or vegetable plate, if eating out
- Salad with fish, chicken, nuts, or avocado
- Baked potato bar with olive oil, broccoli, scallions, sunflower seeds
- Whole avocado and heirloom tomato
- Baked sweet potato with butter, cinnamon, and honey

Snacks/Dips

- Almond butter
- Guacamole
- Hummus
- Sweet Potato Toast
- Sliced green apple with almond or cashew butter
- Raw vegetables with hummus or guacamole
- Boiled egg or deviled eggs (made with GF mayonnaise)
- Carrots and celery sticks

- Berries with slivered almonds
- Nuts—raw almonds, pecans, pistachios, macadamia nuts, or cashews
- Organic popcorn popped on the stove (not microwave popcorn)

Vegetables/Side Dishes

- Arugula Pomegranate Salad
- Asparagus
- Bacon Brussels Sprouts
- Broccoli Slaw
- Coleslaw
- Roasted Root Vegetables
- Roasted Carrots and Parsnips
- Slain Jane Salad
- Sweet Potato Soufflé

Soups

- Homemade Chicken Broth
- Homemade Vegetable Broth
- Black Bean Soup
- White Bean and Cabbage Soup
- Brooke's Chili
- Lentil Soup
- White Chicken Chili
- Mixed Vegetable Soup
- Potato Soup

Dinner

- Chicken and Sautéed Kale
- Chicken Potpie
- Fish Stew
- Lamb Butternut Stew
- Lamb Chops with Plum Sauce
- Meatballs
- Richards' Best Chicken
- Shrimp Stir-fry
- White Bean and Cabbage Soup
- Steak, mushrooms, green beans with slivered almonds, and a salad
- Salmon, sautéed red cabbage, and wild rice
- Baked or grilled chicken, quinoa, and sautéed or grilled zucchini and yellow squash
- Fish, salad, and asparagus
- Beef stew with potato, carrots, celery, bok choy, and onions
- Roasted whole chicken with onions, potatoes, carrots, and bok choy
- Salad with berries, nuts, and seeds

Dessert

- Apple Coconut Cookies
- Baked Pears
- Brownies (Chocolate)
- Coconut Macaroon Cookies
- Dark Chocolate Nut Clusters
- Dark Chocolate Chip Pecan Cookies
- Dark chocolate (at least 70 percent chocolate)
- Dark chocolate–covered strawberries

- One dried date to ten pecans (be careful, as dates are high in sugar)

Bread

- Cornbread
- Corn Pone

Healthy Substitutions

Many unhealthy food choices can be replaced with healthy alternatives that are whole, unprocessed, and naturally GF. The following sections offer several options to replace the gluten-containing foods you eliminated with healthy, flavorful foods.

Sugar Substitutes

Substitute sugar with the natural sweetener stevia, which is an herb. When purchasing stevia, read the ingredients and make sure it does not include a form of sugar such as dextrose or erythritol. Stevia Select™ is a pure, organic stevia extract that contains no fillers, so you only use a small amount. The powder form of stevia is excellent for baking.

Another option is local honey. However, honey raises blood sugar levels, so use it moderately. Also, I found a natural sweetener with zero calories that rates zero on the glycemic index—Lakanto Monkfruit Sweetener (Lakanto.com/); which is made from monk fruit.

In the following list I rank the best natural sugar substitutes based on their glycemic index:

- stevia-0
- monk fruit sweetener-0
- xylitol-12
- agave-15
- coconut sugar-35
- honey-50
- maple syrup-54

Try out these different sweeteners. Choose a natural, low-glycemic sweetener that you can live with and use it sparingly.

Pasta Substitutes

Today you can find many GF variations for pasta. Some natural choices include spaghetti squash, shirataki noodles, or spiralized zucchini. Spaghetti squash can sit on a counter for a couple of weeks, just like a box of spaghetti, and it is simple to cook. Cut it in half, scrape the seeds out of the center, and place it cut side up on a baking sheet with 1/4 inch of water in the pan. Bake at 350°F for 30–40 minutes. When done, scrape the inside with a fork for a low-glycemic "spaghetti." The squash absorbs any flavor you put on it, such as shrimp scampi or spaghetti sauce. This vegetable also tastes great as a side dish with olive oil and seasonings.

To spiralize zucchini, purchase a spiralizer. Push the zucchini through the device and out come your zucchini noodles. For shirataki noodles, cook them as directed on the package and add your sauce. Again, zucchini and shirataki noodles absorb the flavor of the sauce added to them.

Dairy Substitutes

If you have a gluten-related condition, you could also have lactose intolerance. Several healthy dairy substitutes include almond, cashew, and coconut milk. Personally, I enjoy the flavor of toasted coconut almond blend, which combines both of these milks. If you like soy milk, be sure to purchase organic soy products, as soy is one of the Roundup Ready crops that may contain the carcinogen glyphosate.

Follow the Healthy Eating Guidelines

As you prepare your weekly menu, keep in mind these Healthy Eating Guidelines listed below and also in appendix 4:

- Buy organic fruits, vegetables, and meats.
- About 50 percent of your food should be fresh, organic vegetables.
- Eat one fresh, raw serving of a low-glycemic fruit per day. Low-glycemic fruits include green apples, berries, cherries, pears, plums, and grapefruit.
- Do not always eat cooked foods. Eat a couple of servings of raw vegetables every day. Eat a salad for lunch with nuts, meat, or an avocado. When eating out, order a salad or coleslaw as sides since both are raw.
- Plan for 25 percent of your food to be an animal or GF vegetable protein such as beans, nuts, and lean meats. Fish is especially nutritious.
- A variety of different raw nuts and seeds are excellent sources of protein, minerals, and essential fatty acids, and are naturally GF.
- Eat nontraditional grains such as quinoa and amaranth.
- Do not eat sugary cereals. Numerous GF, low-carb breakfast recipes are included in appendix 3.
- Try not to eat anything containing more than 10 grams of sugar in one serving.
- Eat cultured, GF foods such as kimchi and sauerkraut to improve gut health.

When you purchase fewer processed foods, you lower your grocery bill and improve your health and weight.

Prepare to Cook

In my family, as I planned my menu I also designated who would be cooking the meal. I assigned each of my children a night to assist me in the kitchen at least once a week. Mealtime preparation can be a great opportunity for bonding. It is also the perfect time to teach each child about GF cooking and cleaning.

Each morning I checked my menu posted on the refrigerator to determine if I needed to defrost any frozen items. I determined the time to serve our meal and began cooking one hour before that time. Most meals required chopping fresh vegetables, so the extra help was very valuable. When cooking alone, I played music and enjoyed creating a colorful, delicious meal. I felt I was providing my family with a delectable gift.

I always cooked more than what was needed so I would have enough food left over for future meals. If I was taking the time to prepare a healthy meal from scratch, I wanted to make sure my efforts were fully utilized. Everyone served themselves, and the family members who did not assist me in cooking had kitchen clean-up duty.

If you still cook gluten-containing foods, you will need to make sure you do not cross-contaminate with GF items. For example, if you are making a sandwich with regular bread, and another one with a GF bread, do not allow a utensil that touches the regular bread to touch the gluten-free one. Nothing that contains gluten should come into physical contact with food prepared for someone who is GF. In addition, you should utilize excellent cleaning techniques after preparing food that contains gluten.

When eating a GF diet, cooking from scratch is essential to avoid cross-contamination. That is why you cleaned and reorganized your whole kitchen. In addition, use the freshest ingredients you can find. For example, do not buy garlic already minced in a jar. You have no idea how old it is, and it could become contaminated from redipping. Instead, mince a fresh clove of garlic. It might take longer to cook from scratch, but the food will be more nutritious and GF. You will save money by not eating out as much and make fewer trips to the doctor.

Make the transition from eating convenience foods—such as processed foods or eating out—to cooking at home. It doesn't have to be complicated. Create a salad with an avocado or nuts (protein). Load a sliced green apple with GF or homemade almond butter. Blend a fruit smoothie with kale or spinach. Bake a large sweet potato —it is quite filling. Simple meals work just as well as complex dishes.

After you have cooked, store or freeze and label GF and nongluten-free foods. Place them on the appropriate shelves of the refrigerator and freezer. When cleaning up any foods that contained gluten, be sure to toss the sponge or dishtowel in the washer.

Your health is worth the time and effort it takes to master this lifestyle. It took you a lifetime to create your current eating habits, it will take time to break the old habits and reestablish new ones. Choose to put yourself higher on your list of priorities. If you do, you will do a better job of embracing the GF life.

Tips for a Healthier Lifestyle

In addition to embarking on a GF lifestyle, I want to help you improve your overall diet. Can you tell I am a health nut? The following simple tips will help you make healthy lifestyle changes successfully.

Only Eat Until You're Full

As you prepare to eat a healthier GF diet, one positive change you can make is to notice the sensation of fullness as you eat. Some individuals may not be in touch with that feeling anymore. Focus on recognizing when you are full so you do not overeat. You may have to change some of your mealtime habits as well. Eat slowly, chew your food thoroughly, and pay attention to how the food tastes. As you learn to enjoy the taste of foods in their purest form, you'll begin to look for more ways to prepare natural GF meals by using fresh, raw ingredients instead of processed ones.

When you eat processed foods, versus meals you prepare from scratch, it takes a larger quantity of the refined product to fill your stomach because these foods do not contain the original food's fiber. Think of crushing a bag of chips versus shredding carrots and celery. The fresh vegetables will satiate your hunger with a smaller volume. The feeling of fullness stays with you for a longer period too, so you don't need to snack as much. By following this simple lifestyle change, you will eat a smaller quantity of food, but loaded with vitamins, minerals, fiber, and all the nutrients the human body needs.

Pay attention to portion size. Think of your stomach as the size of your fist—before it is stretched out by overeating. Put less food on your plate than you think you will eat. Use a smaller plate. As soon as you feel full, stop eating and put the timer on for five minutes. When the timer rings, you shouldn't feel hungry anymore since it takes a little while for your brain to recognize your stomach reached its capacity. If you stop eating at the first sensation of fullness, in five minutes your brain receptors catch up with the feeling in your stomach.

Recognize you can say no to the voice in your head that demands unhealthy food. Instead of giving in to this voice, put the timer on for fifteen minutes to delay food gratification. Train yourself to wait before you eat so you gain better self-control.

Drink Your Daily Water Intake

If you get hungry in between meals, drink two glasses of water. Water usually curbs the appetite. Most people mistake the feeling of thirst for hunger. Our bodies desperately need water to flush out toxins and prevent dehydration. You also will have more energy when you drink an adequate amount of water.

Other than your caffeinated beverage in the morning, drink only water. Do not drink soft drinks or other unhealthy beverages. If you drink sweet tea and sodas instead of water, this drastically increases your sugar consumption. However, if you are like my daughter, you don't like the taste of water. Choose flavored, carbonated waters on the market that do not contain added sugar or gluten.

The human body is comprised of 75 percent water, and we can't survive for more than a few days without it. Some people think drinking tea, juice, soda, or other drinks will hydrate their body, but they don't. In fact, caffeinated beverages are a diuretic, which causes you to urinate more frequently and lose fluid. Drink an average of eight glasses of water per day.

Your water requirements actually depend upon your weight. Various sources recommend you drink half your weight in ounces every day. Using this formula, a 130-pound person should drink eight glasses of water (130/2 = 65 ounces; 65/8 ounces (1 cup) = 8 glasses).

If you find it challenging to drink eight glasses of water each day, try drinking two glasses of water before breakfast, two before lunch, two midafternoon, and two before dinner.

Try not to consume a lot of water after dinner. Getting up in the middle of the night to go to the bathroom disrupts sleep. Plan when you will consume your eight glasses of water during the day.

Curb Your Sweet Tooth

As you eliminate wheat, sugar, and processed foods from your diet, the craving for sugar may arise. With time your palate changes, and these cravings will lessen. But until then, the following healthy snacks will curb your sweet tooth:

- Slice a green apple, which is low in sugar, and add GF almond or cashew butter to each slice. It tastes sweet;

conversely, the almond butter (recipe in appendix 3) is high in protein. Both the apple and nut butter provide fiber and fill you up.

- Melt 70-percent dark chocolate (GF) in a pan on the stove and add different types of raw nuts until well coated with the chocolate. Place mounds of nut clusters on wax paper. After an hour they harden. Keep in an airtight container on the counter or refrigerator for a week. Nuts contain fiber and are filling.
- Sparingly eat one date along with ten pecan halves. Dates are high in natural sugar, so you only need a smidgen to attain the sweetness. Don't eat too many dates, but instead fill up on the pecans, which are high in protein.
- I grow fruit trees in my yard, so from June through December I pick fresh blueberries, apples, grapes, pears, and oriental persimmons. I eat one serving of fruit each day either for breakfast or as an afternoon snack.
- Curb sweet cravings by adding a teaspoon of raw, unfiltered, unpasteurized apple cider vinegar in a cup of water with a couple drops of stevia.

Surprisingly, taste buds change when you eat natural foods and eliminate wheat, sugar, and processed foods. This change may take from a couple of weeks to months, but it will happen. With time, you will crave the nourishing foods your body needs. Appendix 5 lists these Curb the Sweet Tooth tips for easy reference.

Summary

Learning a new skill is difficult at the beginning, but with time, your new healthy, GF eating habits will become routine. When you take the steps outlined in this chapter, your health improves and symptoms subside. Amber's (chapter 3) migraines and GI symptoms went away completely.

If you need additional support making this lifestyle change, purchase my course, 7 Steps to Reclaim Your Health and Optimal Weight (https://susanuneal.com/courses/7-steps-to-get-off-sugar-and-carbs-course). In this course I help you change your eating habits once and for all.

Healthy foods nourish your body. Continue this lifestyle change for the rest of your life, never turning back to your old eating habits

To assist you with implementing all the tasks from this chapter, I've listed them for you. Take the action steps listed below:

1. Plan your menu for the week and post it on the refrigerator.
2. Create a standardized grocery list that you can print out every week when planning your menu.
3. Go grocery shopping.
4. Prepare healthy GF meals from scratch using the recipes from appendix 3.
5. Pay attention to:
6. Portion control
7. Water intake
8. Use techniques to curb your sweet tooth.

CROSS-CONTAMINATION AND EATING OUT

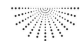

Heather's Story

When Heather worked in New York, she suffered from excruciating abdominal pain and explosive diarrhea. Many times she was not able to leave for work until after her episodes of diarrhea ended. Her boss suggested she be tested for celiac disease because he had a friend who had been recently diagnosed with it.

Heather tried a GF diet for a couple of days, but upon her first taste of lobster bisque she gave up on it. Honestly, she didn't want to stop eating gluten. She lived in a neighborhood with bakeries and restaurants that did not cater to GF clients.

Shortly after that (2010), she went to an allergist. All her food allergy tests were negative. However, her GI symptoms of abdominal pain, bloating, gas, and diarrhea continued.

She read an article that indicated a person needed to be gluten-free for at least a month for symptoms to alleviate. So she tried a GF diet again. Two weeks later her symptoms subsided. She found a bakery in her neighborhood that made one gluten-free item—cupcakes. Every time she needed a delicious snack, she bought one of those.

Years later, while living in California, Heather found it challenging to remain GF. When she cheated on her diet, she experienced headaches. One day, after suffering for three days with an agonizing migraine, she went to see her primary care doctor. He told her that gluten triggered migraines, so he referred her to a gastroenterologist.

Initially, the gastroenterologist ordered a hydrogen breath test to rule out small intestinal bacterial overgrowth (SIBO). She tested positive, and he prescribed antibiotics for the condition. He also indicated that the tests the allergist performed in New York did not rule out celiac disease. To test appropriately for CD, she had to eat gluten for three months.

After eating gluten for ten days, she stopped because of her life-altering GI symptoms. The next time she saw this physician she explained she could not tolerate eating gluten for an extended length of time. The doctor wrote celiac in her chart. Heather doesn't know whether she has celiac disease or non-celiac gluten sensitivity. She never had further testing performed because she could not endure the symptoms associated with eating gluten in order to prepare for the test. Heather's inconclusive diagnosis is similar to my sister Ginny's (from chapter 5).

Currently, Heather owns two restaurants that cater to GF clients. She explained the importance of teaching kitchen staff about cross-contamination with foods containing gluten. "It takes time to educate the kitchen and wait staff. Each person must learn that a utensil, plate, or cooking pan cannot come into contact with food containing gluten if it is being used to prepare a gluten-free menu item."

Since Heather is very sensitive to gluten, she is the perfect person to test all the menu items to ensure they are gluten-free. "Most products I purchase for the restaurant are GF. Condiments are placed in squeeze bottles so gluten contaminated utensils do not come in contact with the food. Bread or gluten-containing foods are only allowed on one portion of the grill. We cook meat in a separate area of the grill."

Heather is a major proponent of the gluten-free movement. She ensures her restaurant patrons have a variety of GF choices. However, she warns, "When eating out you can never be 100 percent positive cross-contamination will not occur if there is gluten in the restaurant."

Just because you eat a gluten-free diet does not mean you cannot enjoy delicious meals at restaurants or attend parties and catered events. Once you master this diet you can go anywhere. This chapter offers suggestions to help you thoroughly enjoy each venue.

The degree of difficulty in eating out correlates with the severity of your sensitivity to gluten. If you have celiac disease or are highly gluten sensitive, like Ginny, eating out can be challenging. Cross-contamination or minuscule amounts of gluten could initiate unpleasant symptoms. If you are wheat sensitive, like me, eating out is easier.

Eating Out

Realistically, you won't be able to prepare your meals at home all the time. With a busy life, some days you are unable to eat at home, so on occasion you will eat out. When you do, you lose control of ensuring that all the ingredients are GF, right down to the seasonings. You are unsure whether the chef or kitchen staff understand cross-contamination. However, you want to enjoy romantic dinners, weddings, conferences, and sporting events. You don't want to be the odd person. When you know how to navigate each venue, you will relax and appreciate the event. Let's first address fast food.

Fast Food

We often use drive-throughs when traveling or in a hurry. Most fast-food restaurants provide a small selection of healthy options to choose from, such as fresh fruit or a salad with raw ingredients. However, dressings pose a problem. You could ask for a GF dressing, but watch out for the high sugar content. Instead, make a homemade salad dressing and carry it with you in a small container. Put it in a resealable bag in case you don't close the lid well and it leaks. Single-serving GF salad dressings, olive oils, and balsamic vinegars are available on the Internet that you can order and carry with you. Ginny asks for a lemon to squeeze on her salads and forgoes the dressing.

Restaurants

Gluten-free dining is common today. Dine at restaurants that serve a large and diverse menu selection, or ones you know provide GF options. Some restaurants display a GF symbol right on the menu for specific items. GF labeling on menus makes selecting your dish easy. However, when you eat at nongluten restaurants, you may encounter issues. Eating out becomes a learning experience. Each time you dine out, you learn from what did and did not work.

Restaurant owner Heather suggests calling the location ahead of time and informing them when a customer with celiac will arrive. This gives the kitchen staff ample time to prepare. Avoid busy hours so you and your meal receive the individual attention you need. If you do not have an opportunity to call ahead of time, speak with the hostess before being seated. Some cooks will come to the table and speak with the individual. It is comforting to know that a restaurant will go out of their way to keep your food free of gluten.

First, check the menu for GF labeling. If a dining establishment does not use GF labeling, verify the ingredients in your meal choice with your waiter. Make sure you ask for your food to be served with no sauces and only salt, pepper, and fresh herbs for seasonings. When your food arrives, assess to make sure it appears to be GF. If your plate comes with a roll, your food is cross-contaminated, so ask for no bread on the plate.

Many restaurants are gluten conscious. When Ginny visited me, she searched the Internet for the top thirty gluten-free restaurants in our area and would only eat at one of those establishments. She did not want to incur gastrointestinal distress while camping in her small travel trailer.

First, she chose Mellow Mushroom, a pizza chain. I wondered how a pizza place could provide GF options with dough being tossed around in the kitchen. Ginny explained that this chain restaurant, and many others, caught on to the GF trend. This establishment creates separate gluten-free kitchen areas for cutting GF pizzas by using dedicated knives, fryers, warming areas, and plates to keep GF food away from gluten-containing ingredients. Separation reduces cross-contamination. They even have vegan cheese for those who are dairy-free. They want satisfied customers to tell their friends about their safe, GF dining experience.

The following chain restaurants provide gluten-free fare:

- Another Broken Egg Café
- Arby's
- BJ's Restaurant and Brewhouse
- Bonefish Grill
- Boston Market
- Burger King
- California Pizza Kitchen
- California Tortilla
- Carrabba's Italian Grill
- Chick-Fil-A
- Chili's Grill & Bar
- Coastal Flats
- Five Guys
- Fogo De Chao
- Jason's Deli
- Jersey Mike's Subs
- Legal Seafood
- Mellow Mushroom
- McDonald's
- Not Your Average Joe's
- PF Chang's China Bistro
- Olive Garden
- On the Border
- Outback Steakhouse

- Pei Wei
- Pieology
- Popeye's Chicken
- Red Robin
- Rodizio Grill
- Ruby Tuesday
- Schlotzsky's Deli
- Seasons 52
- Smash Burger
- Smoothie King
- The Melting Pot
- Wendy's
- Zoe's Kitchen

This diverse selection of restaurants demonstrates the awareness of gluten consciousness in our society. Many chain restaurants list their menus online, which include nutritional information and ingredients. Some restaurants have a separate GF menu. Fast-food places follow standardized guidelines for their ingredients in food preparation. If it is listed as gluten-free, you can usually count on it, unless cross-contamination occurs.

When ordering at other restaurants, Ginny explains to her server that she has a gluten allergy, and eating gluten-free is not a preference but a medical necessity. Even though she does not have celiac disease, she wants to get the point across that she will become ill if her food has any cross-contamination with gluten.

At a recent meal out together, I listened as she explained to the waiter some simple cross-contamination rules. When selecting her entrée, she asked how it was prepared, so she could make an informed decision about ordering it. For example, if it was grilled, she asked if bread was cooked on the same surface. She developed a relationship with the waiter and complimented him when he served her the GF meal. Helping a server understand gluten issues will benefit other gluten-sensitive patrons in the future.

Don't be embarrassed to ask for your food to be gluten-free; even people without dietary restrictions ask for special considerations. If you are dining at a restaurant that has GF-labeled food on the menu, you do not need to ask the following questions. However, when Ginny dines at restaurants that do not have GF menu items, she asks her server the following specific questions regarding food preparation:

- How is the food prepared? (grilled, sautéed, baked)
- What seasonings are used? Are they certified gluten-free?
- Is the dish marinated? Does the marinade contain soy or gluten?
- Does the dish contain a sauce? What are the ingredients of the sauce?
- Was the food prepared on a griddle or grill that also was used for cooking bread?
- Is there a separate fryer for gluten-free foods?
- Does the salad dressing contain gluten or soy?
- Are the hash browns made from fresh potatoes?
- Is the bacon real or artificial?
- Does the egg mixture for omelets contain wheat? Is the mix from a box, or is the omelet made from real eggs?
- Do you use separate utensils and pans for cooking GF foods?

Ginny embraced the GF lifestyle several years ago, so she knows the right questions to ask. As you educate yourself, you will learn which questions to ask too. Sometimes the chef comes out of the kitchen and speaks with Ginny. Most restaurants gladly accommodate her requests to eat gluten-free. Today it is no longer challenging to find excellent GF establishments. I can't imagine the difficulty of navigating the gluten-free lifestyle a couple of decades ago. When word spreads that a restaurant serves safe, GF foods, it increases their business. Praise and tip your waiter well for accommodating your dietary requests.

On some occasions you may not be able to choose the restaurant, and the one you are eating at may not accommodate GF customers. Numerous menu options are naturally gluten-free, or the chef can adapt a recipe to make it gluten-free. Salads are an excellent choice, and you can ask for oil and vinegar instead of a premade salad dressing and no croutons. But first, ask your waiter if the salad dressing is labeled as GF. Manufacturers are catching on to the trend. Hidden Valley® is one company that has certified GF dressings. Heather only purchases GF dressings for her restaurants.

If the waiter does not seem to understand the GF food preparation process, you can ask to speak with the chef. Sometimes cooks like to mingle with their guests, especially if it is not a busy time for the restaurant. Chefs learn about gluten-free dietary accommodations in culinary school. You may provide an opportunity for him to put his skills and knowledge to work.

Go online to search for the top thirty GF restaurants in your area. These restaurants catered to Ginny's dietary needs perfectly. With today's technology, information is at your fingertips.

If you're unsure whether a particular location has GF items, call and ask at a time when the establishment is not busy. They could send you a copy of the menu if it is not available online. In time you'll figure out which local restaurants, as well as chains, prepare delicious GF meals. For me, it is Heather's restaurant. It's right down the road from my house, and she serves gluten-free cocktails. If you dine at local restaurants that don't serve GF menu items, suggest they carry some. The chef and owner may be excited to accommodate your request and broaden their menu. Spread the word about your exceptional GF dining experience with family and friends.

If you receive a meal that contains gluten, return it. Obvious examples include croutons on the salad or a roll on your plate. Don't eat something that will make you sick. You are paying good money for food, and you deserve for it to be gluten-free. When asking for your meal to be remade, keep the original food served with you at the table while the restaurant staff prepares your replacement so the staff does not merely remove the gluten-containing item. Instead, they should replace the entire dish.

Gluten-free dining-out cards are available on the Internet. You can download and print them out. These cards contain a clear description of the food and preparation methods necessary to ensure you receive a GF meal. Give your server a card to explain your dietary specifications. These dining cards are available in different languages so you can take them with you when traveling. You may want to laminate a card and carry paper versions to give to waiters and chefs.

Another healthy living tip will help you not overeat. At some restaurants the serving size may be substantial. Therefore, when served a large plate of food, before you begin eating, determine how much you will consume at this meal to prevent overeating. You might even ask for a to-go container at the beginning of your meal to store what you will not eat at this meal. It is difficult to stop unless you establish boundaries before you begin eating delicious foods.

Catered Events

Are you looking forward to attending a wedding, conference, or party? Usually you choose from two options for the main course. Many items include delicious sauces that most likely contain gluten. However, you can navigate the limited menu for these catered events.

First, call the catering company directly and see if they provide GF options. There is probably more than one person attending who has a gluten-related disorder, since one out of every ten people is affected. The catering company may accommodate your request. During the event explain to your waiter that you spoke with the company and ordered a GF menu selection.

Unfortunately, often the servers at catered events are unfamiliar with the type of food served and whether it contains gluten. It's not like a restaurant where the waiter is familiar with the food and can correctly answer your concerns. Therefore, calling the caterer before the event is your best bet to attaining a GF meal. Your host for any event should be able to give you the caterer's information.

The second tactic used to navigate catered events is to eat before you go so you won't be hungry. Focus on having fun at the event instead of eating. If you do eat, be choosy in selecting GF items. You can always eat fresh vegetables, fruits, and cheese, but avoid the dips as they usually contain gluten. You could also take a bag of nuts to munch on along with your fruit and veggies.

The nuts at catered events may contain gluten if they are seasoned, sugared, or coated. Vegetables and meats that do not include a sauce may be gluten-free. If you call the catering company, you can also ask about any seasonings they use. Seasonings were my sister's most frequent gluten culprit.

Buffets

Numerous events use buffets to offer a large selection of food. If possible, assess the food in the buffet before you get in line. Determine what appears to be GF and load up on those items. Salads and plain vegetables are a wise choice. If staff is available, ask what foods are GF. If they do not know, ask if the spice used on the vegetables contains gluten. When placing food on your plate, be sure to take a portion of an undisturbed section of each buffet item to avoid cross-contamination. A guest may have used a serving utensil from a gluten-containing buffet item to scoop food out of the GF dish.

Dinner Guest

It's always fun to be a dinner guest at someone's home. However, now that you're eating GF, this adds challenges. Call the person hosting the event and politely explain that it is medically necessary for you to eat a gluten-free diet. Otherwise, you will experience unpleasant symptoms. Most people are receptive to discussing the menu with you and accommodating your dietary request. You could also provide GF suggestions for the host's menu and even ask if you could bring a dish. If the menu can't be modified, suggest bringing a few things for yourself.

Also, explain about cross-contamination, such as redipping in a condiment or using the same spatula to serve gluten and nongluten foods. Most people are unaware of cross-contamination. Tell your host that you are delighted to be invited, and having fun and socializing at this event is more important to you than eating.

Eat a snack before you attend the dinner in case there are items you cannot eat. You don't want to be starving and tempted to eat food that contains gluten. When serving yourself, take larger portions of the foods you can eat, such as salads, plain vegetables, and meat. That way your plate does not look empty. Avoid casseroles and anything with a gravy or sauce. Watch out for cross-contamination during the dinner. You don't need to point this out to others, but be diligent for yourself.

Thank your host for accommodating your dietary needs. He or she did not have to make an effort. From time to time, even your closest friends and family members will forget about your gluten issue and serve foods that are not gluten-free. They don't forget or make mistakes because they don't care about you. It's hard to juggle their life and remember your issues as well. Also, sometimes people do not understand the GF diet, especially when it comes to cross-contamination. Or they didn't realize a specific spice or sauce contained gluten. It's hard for you to understand all the different foods that contain gluten, imagine how hard it may be for people who don't deal with a gluten disorder.

Pot Lucks

Bring a delicious dish or two of your own. Assess the food selection before getting in line. Be selective about what you eat because you don't know what is in it. Although, if you know who made the dish, feel free to ask. Serve yourself a large portion size of your dish along with plain salads and raw fruits and vegetables. You could also snack before you get there or eat something more filling when you get home.

Sporting Events/Concerts

Whether you're at a concert or a college football game, menu options are dismal. Plan to bring all the snacks you need to last for the whole event. If you can't bring a snack because of arena or stadium restrictions, ask the attendant at the concession stand if the popcorn is labeled as GF, as some anticaking agents in popcorn salt may contain gluten.

Conferences/Business Meetings

Conferences and business meetings are similar to eating at catered events. Assess the food provided. Eat the salad and add your own dressing and nuts if you brought them. Again, preplanning is essential.

Bakery

Bakeries can be hazardous because wheat flour can stay airborne for hours after a baker manipulates the flour. The airborne particles could contaminate surfaces (countertops, cabinet handles) and any uncovered GF products. If you have celiac disease or a wheat allergy, avoid bakeries, or find a GF bakery.

Traveling

When traveling, preplanning is essential. Whether traveling by plane or car, be sure to carry your own GF snacks to get you through the trip in case you do not find any GF menu options. Restaurant chains that cater to GF dining are excellent choices.

If you're flying, and you ordered a gluten-free meal, be sure to check with the flight attendant. Explain that you are supposed to receive a GF menu item. After the meal arrives, make sure it appears to be GF. If you are suspicious because of sauces or a roll, eat the snack you brought with you instead. It's better to be safe than sorry, especially on a plane. In airports, you can usually find fruits or salads that are naturally GF at kiosks; again avoid the dressing, unless single-serve GF dressings are available. Large airports have restaurant chains that carry GF items.

Cruise lines accommodate dietary restrictions. They prefer you contact them in advance of your sail date so they can order a larger quantity of GF items. Once onboard, speak with the ship's maître d, who will explain your GF dining venue options. If you forget to notify the cruise line ahead of time, talk with the maître d once on board. You can still eat GF, but the menu may be limited. Eating GF during your cruise should be a positive experience.

When staying at a hotel, the concierge desk should know which local restaurants provide gluten-free options. They can even make your reservation. For extended stays, plan for a kitchenette in your hotel room, condo, or Airbnb so you can prepare some of your meals. A microwave and small refrigerator will make your trip easier. You can purchase a heat-resistant toaster bag and insert your GF piece of bread. That way you can use a toaster at hotels and other lodging establishments. When you need to purchase foods at a grocery store you're not familiar with, be sure to read the food labels to verify the ingredients.

Larger cities provide more GF restaurant options. The same goes for traveling on the west coast of the US. This area is much more adept regarding the dietary needs of patrons. Use Ginny's trick and search the Internet for the top thirty gluten-free restaurants in the cities you will visit. Call restaurants before you go to ensure they can accommodate your dietary requests.

Also, research grocery stores, markets, and fast-food places in the area you will be staying. If you find a health food store close to your destination, call them to ask about any GF items they carry. You may be able to pick up healthy GF snacks at these stores.

When traveling to foreign countries, gluten-free labeling laws vary. Therefore you cannot count on the labeling of items like in the United States. Consequently, it would be prudent to learn foreign language words for bread, gluten, and similar foods. Print out dining cards in the native language of the country you will visit. You can hand your server a card at each restaurant. European countries are more familiar with the GF diet.

Some tour groups and cruise lines cater to GF travelers. If you choose to use one of these, your dietary needs should be met. Online celiac disease support groups may also provide tips and advice regarding restaurants and lodging.

Setbacks

When symptoms return, you were probably exposed to gluten. Sometimes it's hard to figure out exactly what you ingested that triggered the reaction. Keep a list of potential gluten culprits in your journal or the notes app of your phone. If symptoms return, check your list to verify if you previously suspected the food item. For example, once I cooked a meal using two different GF spices. Unfortunately, my daughter experienced gastrointestinal distress from the dinner. I determined that the double dose of 20 ppm of each gluten-free spice was too much for her. Therefore, I do not use more than one GF spice when cooking. This is part of the learning curve in solving the gluten puzzle.

When Ginny first started the GF diet, every time she sat down to eat something different she researched whether the food contained gluten. Becoming GF is a learning experience. One you figure out all the foods that contain gluten, simply avoid them.

Two years into Ginny's gluten-free journey she ate an anniversary dinner with her husband at a fancy restaurant. She enjoyed salmon that the restaurant claimed was GF. Unfortunately, the seasonings must have contained gluten or else there was cross-contamination in the kitchen. As a result, when Ginny got home she was in bed for three hours (no, not with her husband) with excruciating abdominal pain and diarrhea. She treated her pain with a heating pad. It felt as though someone punched her in the stomach. After that experience, when eating out she only orders meat and vegetables seasoned with salt, pepper, and fresh herbs. Otherwise, she fears eating or drinking something that contains gluten and experiencing gastrointestinal distress. Even if you call the restaurant or caterer, gluten contamination may still occur from time to time. Learn from each new experience.

Temptations

In addition to a physical setback from eating hidden sources of gluten, there are setbacks from temptations to eat gluten-containing foods. Many people get into a cycle of diets. They do well for a while, but when they make a mistake, they feel terrible about themselves, as if they have failed. So they give up and return to unhealthy eating habits. An all-or-nothing attitude is perilous. Just because you slipped doesn't mean you should give up. As with any attempt to improve your life, when you stumble, get up and try again.

It is important to determine what is causing your desire to cheat on your GF diet. In my faith-based book *7 Steps to Get Off Sugar and Carbohydrates*, I review the three most common reasons we are tempted to cheat: food addiction, Candida overgrowth in the GI tract, or unhealthy emotional connection with food.

Sometimes we lie to ourselves by saying, "Just this once," "I need this comfort food," "It's a special occasion," or "It won't hurt me." The list of excuses can go on and on. The key to saying no is understanding the consequences to your health.

Sometimes the negative health issue does not occur within a few hours or even days, so you don't realize the damage it does to your body. If you continue to cheat, it could have severe effects on your health.

I have seven small nodules on my thyroid. The doctor says they are within normal limits so he will monitor them. But thyroid nodules are not normal! Hashimoto's disease, an autoimmune disorder that affects the thyroid, may be triggered by a gluten intolerance. I need to avoid wheat to prevent the adverse effects it causes my body—results I do not see, feel, or realize at the time.

To help you with your resolve, make a list of the top five benefits you experience when implementing the GF diet. Now make a list of the top five consequences of eating gluten or wheat. Keep both lists on your refrigerator and look at them when you are tempted to cheat. Renew your mind and focus on longevity and quality of life. Join an online support group to find the support you need. People who have social support groups are more likely to stick to the GF diet. To manage your sweet tooth, check out appendix 5 for a list of sweet healthy snacks. Appendix 3 also contains several healthy GF dessert recipes.

Food Addiction

We need to understand that sugar and wheat are addictive. Addiction is a compulsive repetition of an activity despite life-damaging consequences. Food addiction is a biochemical disorder that cannot be controlled by willpower alone. If you have not considered the possibility of having a food addiction, do not feel shame over the terminology. Your body has fallen prey to the accumulative effects of sugar and wheat that are ingrained in so many of our culture's food habits. The surgeon general's 2016 report indicated that addiction is a chronic brain disease, not a moral failing.[1]

Two hallmarks of addiction include persistent desire and repeated unsuccessful attempts to stop. Being addicted to food is like having an alien inside of you who takes control of your body and eats a bunch of unhealthy food. You can't stop it. Sugar and wheat hijack your body. You can't halt the craving or binges no matter what diet or method you try. Your willpower is never enough. Understanding that food addiction is not a lack of self-control but a rewiring of the brain helps you have more compassion for yourself.

How does addiction happen? Foods containing sugar and wheat

cause the release of an excess amount of dopamine in the brain. Dopamine, a feel-good neurohormone, releases when we eat foods high in sugar, take opiate drugs, smoke cigarettes, drink alcohol, cuddle with our kids, pet a dog, or enjoy sex.[2] A dopamine rush can rewire the brain to desire more of whatever causes its release. Therefore, when a food addict sees sugary foods, dopamine releases and causes the person's focus to narrow.[3] She can think only about eating that food item to experience the euphoria it brings.

Scientists found that the part of the brain that restrains behavior (self-control) was abnormally quiet in rats with an addiction. Unfortunately, when we struggle with the desire for unhealthy foods, the part of the brain that inhibits addictive behavior becomes silent, and we lose the ability to have self-control.[4]

One of the worst carbohydrate culprits is wheat because a polypeptide in wheat crosses the blood-brain barrier, which separates the bloodstream from the brain, and binds to the brain's morphine receptors.[5] Opiate drugs (morphine, codeine, heroin, cocaine) bind to these same receptors.

During this journey of change, learn from your mistakes. Have you ever told yourself, "I'll take one bite and that will satisfy my sugar craving"? If so, you understand that logic never works. You can't take only one bite, because dopamine releases in the brain and causes a physiological response that your self-control cannot manage.

Even before you take the first bite, if you desire the food, dopamine secretes in the brain. Scientists proved this through MRI imaging of the brains of addicts. Therefore, when you feel the temptation to eat wheat-containing carbohydrates, recognize it. If you understand what is going on in your brain, you can more effectively fight the temptation.

Determining whether you are a food addict will help you understand yourself and enable you to overcome this addiction effectively. Use these links to online quizzes to determine if you are addicted to food: foodaddicts.org/am-i-a-food-addict and oa.org/newcomers/how-do-i-start/are-you-a-compulsive-overeater/.

The first step in dealing with any addiction is to acknowledge it.

Even if you don't see yourself this way, understanding your body's reaction to foods is crucial for making improvements in your diet and feeling the benefits of a healthier approach to food. If you discover that you are a food addict, take the steps necessary to begin to overcome this to improve your lifestyle and food habits.

Addiction rewires the neural circuits in a person's brain. Therefore, the brain assigns a higher value to sugar and wheat than other foods. Subliminal food cues excite the brain's reward system and contribute to a relapse. People fall prey to these unseen triggers. That is why it is imperative to identify what sets off your desire and eliminate the trigger. Similarly, an alcoholic should not go into a bar. As your health improves from eating a GF diet, you cannot let down your guard. Recognizing you have a food addiction and avoiding the triggers will keep you in recovery mode and allow you to maintain this healthier lifestyle.

If you are a food addict and are not able to stop the cycle of addiction, my faith-based book *Christian Study Guide for 7 Steps to Get Off Sugar and Carbohydrates* can help you start on the path to recovery.

Plan for Pitfalls

Changing the way you eat is a challenging journey, but one you can conquer. Every morning, determine your menu for the day and what temptations you might encounter. What time of the day would you most likely engage in unhealthy eating? Decide how you will fight food temptation for that specific day.

When you recognize temptation, remove yourself from the area containing the food, and record the trigger in your journal. Also, write down five reasons why you do not want to eat the food. Put the timer on for ten minutes and distract yourself. Some strategies for resisting temptation include: go for a walk, call a friend, drink two glasses of water, or lean on your faith, whatever that might be. Also, focus on how far you have come with embracing the GF lifestyle.

If you relapse, get up, brush the dust off yourself, and start again. Realize what triggered your cravings. Was it your emotions? In your journal, keep track of what you ate, why you ate it, what triggered you to eat it, and what you might do the next time you are tempted.

Were you tempted by something you saw on TV? If yes, don't watch the commercials. Was it food someone else in your family ate? If yes, ask them not to eat it in front of you. Ask them to store all tempting food products out of your sight. Through journaling, you can identify your triggers and strategize how to avoid them. It is normal for people to stay the course and then fall off the wagon. This cycle continues to repeat itself, but as you continue you will gain control of your body and mind and ultimately experience victory.

Thought Life

Our thought life can sabotage our success. We must change our thought process from negativity and despair to positivity and hope if we want to succeed in making the GF lifestyle changes necessary for a healthy future. We are far from perfect. Improvement is the correct mind-set to succeed. Replace any negativity about yourself with grace.

A way to think of grace is to consider how you would advise your best friend who calls you after she has binged on food. You would show her grace and encourage her to start again. When you mess up, think about what you would tell her. Don't be so hard on yourself. Understand that at some point you will eat unhealthy gluten-containing foods. Expect it, acknowledge it, and move on.

This lifestyle change is not an all-or-nothing situation. If you don't follow the GF diet 100 percent of the time, don't think of it as failure. You cannot change your eating habits overnight. Don't get discouraged when you do not meet your expectations. Making this lifestyle change is difficult, but you can succeed.

Let Your Mistakes Motivate You

As your diet improves, when you eat foods containing wheat, sugar, or refined gluten-containing carbohydrates, you will feel sluggish. You may not even feel like getting out of bed the next day, and you will probably be foggy brained. Remember the way you feel when you eat clean GF foods. This should motivate you to eat GF.

Every time I slip, I pay for it the next day, and that motivates me to eat healthier. I like waking up feeling energized and ready to start my day, rather than feeling groggy. That way, I can do anything to the best of my ability. When you eat poorly, recognize it. Choose to eat better for the rest of that day. Tomorrow is a new day, and with it comes new hope and a fresh resolve.

Summary

It's normal to worry about eating away from home. You might feel like people are staring at you during an event when you are not eating what everyone else is eating or when you use your own salad dressing. Don't let these feelings of not fitting in stop you from attending social events. With practice and patience you can handle these challenges.

Whether you are dealing with a food addiction or not, as you nourish your body with proper nutrients, it will begin to heal itself of diabetes, hypertension, headaches, allergies, skin problems, joint pain —the list goes on. Complete healing will take time, though some symptoms may disappear right away. You will lose weight without starving yourself too. Your mental clarity and speed of thought processes will improve. You will love the new you!

It is vital to gain knowledge about living gluten-free. Join a blog such as celiac.org and read up on other people's experiences. This helped Ginny understand how to eat GF in many different circumstances. Making wise GF food choices goes hand-in-hand with your knowledge about the subject.

Don't focus on the things you can't eat but the things you can. Your old comfort foods were probably the items that brought you discomfort. Instead, choose new favorites. Within the first few months of embracing the gluten-free lifestyle, you should experience significant improvements in the quality of your life. Rejoice in your newfound health!

APPENDIX 1: SUSAN'S HEALTH
CRISIS

I combated a health crisis at the age of forty-nine. In November of that year, I had a crown placed on a tooth. Little did I know that this event would mark the beginning of the loss of my good health. Over the following nine months, that tooth abscessed and poisoned my body, resulting in ten different medical diagnoses.

One month after the crown, I began having two menstrual cycles every month. The double periods continued, and eventually, fifteen months later, I had surgery to remove two uterine polyps.

Two months later I experienced depression and craved chocolate. Where I used to eat a couple of candy bars per year, now I binged on Ghirardelli chocolate every evening.

In March I was diagnosed with an ovarian cyst, and two months later, adrenal fatigue. Although exhausted, I had difficulty sleeping. By this point I should have known something was wrong with my body. Nevertheless, I didn't realize the severity of my physical problems even though as a yoga instructor I taught my clients to be in tune with their bodies.

My doctor prescribed three different adrenal vitamins five times a day for my adrenal fatigue. That's fifteen vitamin pills per day! The physician also prescribed progesterone cream for the ovarian cyst and hormonal imbalance, as I was experiencing perimenopause. That summer I was so exhausted that I could not attend my aunt's funeral because I did not have the stamina to fly across the country. Even my husband and children did not understand how depleted I felt.

In July I saw flashes of light in my left eye when I quickly turned my head to the left. Two months later I was diagnosed with a hole in my retina. Retinal tears can lead to blindness if the retina becomes detached.

In August I began experiencing visual migraines even though I had never suffered from headaches. That month I went to my dentist for a cleaning and told my hygienist I felt a bump above one of my teeth. She informed me that was not a good sign, and the dentist discovered that the tooth I had crowned in November had abscessed and drained its putrid fluid into my gastrointestinal system. I still didn't realize that the effects of my abscessed tooth likely caused all the other symptoms.

I had an emergency root canal along with ten days of antibiotics and two weeks of steroids. Afterward, I was so fatigued I could not even put away the groceries after shopping. No one understood how depleted my system was because on the outside I looked fine, but on the inside, I was a train wreck.

In September my doctor found I was anemic and low in vitamin D, so he told me to take iron and vitamin D supplements. He also referred me to an optometrist for the flashes of light in my eye. The optometrist performed emergency laser surgery to prevent a detached retina. When I turn my head sharply to the left, I still have a flash of light, and I will never regain that part of my vision.

In the fall my health further declined. I felt utterly drained and sick all the time, and I could have easily stayed in bed. However, my family needed me. My doctors were unable to do much for me except recommend vitamin D, iron supplements, adrenal vitamins, and progesterone cream. So I began alternative health-care therapies such as massage, acupuncture, and colonic irrigation.

Through a colonic irrigation, the therapist found a candida infection in my colon. I had never heard of this type of infection before, despite being an RN, since candidiasis (candida infection from a Candida fungus) of the gut is not taught in mainstream medicine. Even my internal medicine doctor didn't know how to rid me of this yeast infection in my intestine.

A candida infection in your colon is similar to a vaginal yeast infection. Women are prone to these when they take antibiotics because the drug kills off beneficial flora in a person's body. I had recently taken both antibiotics and a steroid.

I turned fifty that August and lost my health. For five decades, I took my good health for granted. Now I realized it was precious. Ultimately, what occurred in my body originated from an abscessed tooth and resulted in ten different medical diagnoses in the following order:

1. Bimonthly periods caused by uterine polyps
2. Depression
3. Ovarian cyst
4. Adrenal fatigue
5. Hormonal imbalance
6. Retinal tear
7. Visual migraine
8. Anemia
9. Low vitamin D level
10. Candidiasis infection of my colon

My colonic therapist gave me a copy of *The Body Ecology Diet* by Donna Gates so I could educate myself. The information in this book confirmed I had an overgrowth of Candida in my gastrointestinal system. I followed a strict anti-Candida diet to get rid of the infection.

Candida feeds off of carbohydrates. Therefore, a physical component of my craving for sugar and carbs was an overgrowth of this harmful microorganism. Having candidiasis is like having a monster take control of your appetite. If you want to determine if you have a candida overgrowth in your gut, take the Candida Quiz at Candi-Quiz.com.If you want to determine if you have a candida overgrowth in your gut, take the Candida Quiz at CandiQuiz.com.

I fought this culprit and restored my gut flora. The gut flora consists of beneficial microorganisms (also known as probiotics) that strengthen the immune system and defend against unfriendly bacteria and pathogens that cause disease.

For the following eight months, I struggled to regain my health. To eradicate the Candida, I stopped eating fruit, rice, flour, sugar, and desserts. I lost a lot of weight. During this time, I took one step forward and two steps back, then three steps forward and one step back. It was a slow process, but after eight months on this strict diet, I finally regained my health.

I felt healed. The diet required great self-control, but I was determined to succeed because I desperately wanted my health back. Ultimately I beat the candida infection in my colon and restored my adrenal glands. We have glorious bodies that will heal themselves if we give them the right building blocks.

APPENDIX 2: RESOURCES

1. The Celiac Disease Foundation website Celiac.org
2. Beyond Celiac at BeyondCeliac.org
3. The Celiac Disease and Gluten-Free Diet website Celiac.com
4. The National Celiac Association website NationalCeliac.org
5. At-home blood test kits available through https://imaware.health/celiac-disease/at-home-blood-test/
6. Genetic tests (Human Leukocyte Antigen—HLA–DQ2 and HLA–DQ8) available through https://blog.23andme.com/health-traits/new-23andme-report-celiac-disease/
7. Raising Our Celiac Kids (ROCK), part of the National Celiac Association: RaisingOurCeliacKids.org/
8. For GF grocery items: GlutenFreeMall.com at GlutenfreeMall.com/catalog/
9. Gluten-Free Living at Glutenfreeliving.com/
10. A gluten intolerance online group at gluten.org/
11. The Gluten-Free Casein-Free Diet at gfcfdiet.com/
12. Food addiction online quizzes at

https://www.foodaddicts.org/am-i-a-food-addict and https://oa.org/newcomers/how-do-i-start/are-you-a-compulsive-overeater/

APPENDIX 3: RECIPES

I am excited to feature several grain-free, sugar-free, and hunger-free recipes by Melissa Monroe McGehee. Her cookbooks *Satisfying Eats* and *Comforting Eats* offer delicious meal options so you can cook and enjoy your favorite recipes without grains yet not feel deprived. For more information on her cookbooks and recipes, visit Satisfying-Eats.com.

A healthy change when baking it to eliminate sugar. Stevia is an excellent sugar substitute. You can find baking stevia in grocery stores or online. Stevia Select™ is a pure stevia extract with no fillers and is Melissa's preference for baking. Be careful, it only takes a small amount to sweeten dishes. Other great sweeteners include honey, maple syrup, agave, xylitol, coconut sugar, and monk fruit sugar.

If you are lactose intolerant, like me, you can substitute the butter with ghee (clarified butter) in these recipes. Nondairy yogurts made from coconuts or almonds are a substitute for sour cream. When purchasing meats, buy grass-fed, organic meats that were not given hormones and antibiotics. I purchase organic vegetables if they have a thin skin or are on the Environmental Working Group's (EWG) Dirty Dozen list. I post this list each year on my Healthy Living Series Facebook group at https://www.facebook.com/HealthyLivingSeries/.

Please join the group to learn healthy living tips to improve your health and well-being.

I always purchase organic strawberries, peaches, plums, apple, beets, cucumbers, salad greens, tomatoes, and potatoes as they are thin-skinned. I do not want to ingest the herbicides and insecticides sprayed on produce. If a vegetable or fruit has a thick skin, I usually don't buy organic, such as avocados and winter squashes. These skins are usually peeled and not consumed.

BREAKFAST

Avocado Egg Bake

(Makes 2 servings)
2 large avocados, firm
4 eggs

Preheat the oven to 400°F. Be sure to use large avocados; small ones will not accommodate the egg. Cut avocado in half lengthwise and place on a baking sheet. Do not peel. Remove the avocado pit, and scoop out a little bit of avocado so a cracked egg will fit inside the pit hole. Crack an egg into each avocado half. Bake for 20–25 minutes depending upon how done you like your eggs.

Bacon, Lettuce, Scrambled Eggs

(Makes 3 servings)
Butterhead/Buttercrunch lettuce
Half a package bacon
6 eggs
2 avocados, diced
2 tablespoons olive oil
¼ teaspoon salt
1/8 teaspoon pepper
1 tablespoon fresh parsley

Place butterhead lettuce leaves on plates. Fry bacon and crumble into pieces on lettuce. Scramble eggs in oil along with seasonings. Place on top of the bacon. Chop avocados and put on top of eggs.

Bacon-Wrapped Green Apples

(Makes 3 servings)
Half a package bacon
3 green apples

Wash apples and slice with an apple corer/slicer. Fry bacon just until done. Then wrap each piece around a slice of apple. Hold bacon in place with a toothpick.

Banana Quinoa Oatmeal

(Makes 4 servings)
1 cup of quinoa cooked in 2 cups of water (about 4 cups cooked)
2 smashed slightly green bananas (lower in sugar if green)
¾ cup chopped walnuts
1 teaspoon cinnamon
1 teaspoon vanilla
1 tablespoon honey or 1 teaspoon of stevia
¾ cup almond or coconut milk

In a large pot, add water and bring it to a boil. Add the quinoa, turn down to low heat, cover and cook for 20 minutes. Smash bananas and chop walnuts. Combine the rest of the ingredients with the cooked quinoa on stovetop and warm.

Berry Smoothie

(Makes 1 serving)
1 cup frozen berries (any type)
1 cup fresh spinach leaves
3/4 cup coconut or almond milk

Mix all ingredients in a blender. Add ice cubes to thicken.

Eggs Benedict
(Makes 2 servings)
1 tomato, sliced (instead of English muffin)
4 eggs
4 slices of bacon or ham
Spinach leaves, raw
1 avocado, sliced

Place two thick slices of tomato per plate. Add a few spinach leaves to the top of each tomato slice. Fry bacon and place on sliced tomato. Fry eggs in bacon grease and put on top of the bacon. Top with sliced avocado.

Sauce
½ cup butter or ghee
3 egg yolks
1 tablespoon fresh lemon juice
1/8 teaspoon salt

In a saucepan, melt butter over medium heat. In a bowl, whisk egg yolks, lemon, and salt. Over medium heat, slowly pour the egg mixture into the melted butter while stirring with a whisk. The sauce should thicken in a few minutes. Pour on top of avocado.

Mushroom Frittata
(Makes 4 servings)
1 bunch of scallions, diced
1 bag of spinach
1 container of mushrooms, diced
6 eggs
2 tablespoons olive oil
1 clove garlic, minced
1 teaspoon fresh thyme
¼ teaspoon salt
1/8 teaspoon pepper

Preheat the oven to 425°F. In a bowl, beat the eggs and seasonings together. Slice the scallions and mushrooms. Heat the oil in a cast-iron skillet over medium heat. Add the scallions and mushrooms, stirring often. After five minutes, add spinach and garlic, stirring for a couple of minutes. Pour egg mixture into sautéed vegetables. Stir the vegetables and eggs until well combined. Transfer the cast-iron skillet to the oven for five minutes or until eggs are well done.

Omelet
(Makes 4 servings)
6 eggs
1 bunch of scallions, diced
2 cups spinach, raw
1 cup mushrooms, diced
½ red bell pepper, diced
2 tablespoons olive oil
1 tablespoon fresh parsley
¼ teaspoon salt
¼ teaspoon pepper

In a bowl, beat the eggs and seasonings together. Dice the scallions, bell pepper, and mushrooms. Heat the oil in a skillet over medium heat. Add the diced vegetables, stirring often. After five minutes, add egg mixture. Stir the vegetables and eggs until well combined. Cook on low heat until eggs are firm.

Prosciutto-Wrapped Pears
(Makes 3 servings)
3 pears, firm
1 package of prosciutto
Fresh mint

Wash and slice pears with an apple corer/slicer. Wrap each slice of pear with prosciutto, adding a fresh mint leaf to the center. Hold prosciutto in place with a toothpick.

Spinach-Topped Eggs
  (Makes 1 serving)
  1 cup spinach, raw
  2 eggs
  ½ avocado, sliced
  2 tablespoons olive oil
  Salt (to taste)
  Pepper (to taste)
  Paprika (to taste)

Place freshly washed spinach on a plate. Fry two eggs in oil; place on top of spinach. Add seasonings and avocado to the eggs.

Poultry Patties
  (Makes 8 servings)
  2 pounds ground turkey or chicken (make sure it is gluten-free)
  ½ bunch scallions, diced
  4 cloves garlic, minced
  2 teaspoons sage
  3/4 teaspoon salt
  3 tablespoons olive oil

Slice the scallions and mix by hand with the ground poultry, garlic, and seasonings. Heat olive oil in a skillet and cook the patties on medium heat for 7–10 minutes on each side until completely done.

BREAKFAST BREADS

Apple Quinoa Breakfast Muffins
  (Makes 8 servings)
  1 cup cooked quinoa
  ½ cup applesauce
  1 mashed banana (lower in sugar if green)
  ½ cup almond or coconut milk
  1 tablespoon honey or maple syrup

2 teaspoons baking stevia or sweetener of choice, to taste
1 teaspoon vanilla extract
1 teaspoon cinnamon
2½ cups GF oats
1 apple, finely chopped

Preheat the oven to 375°F. Grease a muffin pan with olive oil. In a bowl, smash the slightly green banana. Add wet ingredients to bowl and mix with a spoon. Combine rest of the ingredients, leaving the apple for last. Pour ingredients into muffin tins. Bake for 20–25 minutes or until a toothpick inserted into the center comes out clean.

Blueberry-Lemon Muffins
  From Melissa Monroe McGehee's blog Satisfyingeats.com
  (Makes 8 muffins; 6 grams of carbs per muffin)
  1 cup plus 2 tablespoons almond flour
  2 tablespoons ground flaxseed (or extra almond flour)
  2 tablespoons coconut flour
  1½ teaspoons baking soda
  ½ teaspoon Stevia Select™ or sweetener of choice, to taste
  2 tablespoons salted butter or coconut oil, melted
  3 eggs, well beaten
  1½ teaspoons vanilla extract
  1 tablespoon plus 1 teaspoon lemon juice
  Zest of one lemon
  1/3 cup sour cream or nondairy plain yogurt
  2/3 cup fresh blueberries
  Optional toppings: chopped pecans or unsweetened shredded coconut

Preheat the oven to 350°F. Grease or line muffin tins. In a medium bowl, mix dry ingredients. Add everything else except blueberries and mix well. Taste for sweetness and lemon flavor; adjust if needed. Gently fold in blueberries. Don't overmix the batter or it will turn blue. Portion out the dough into 8 muffin tins. Bake for

20–25 minutes until a toothpick inserted into the center comes out clean.

Cinnamon Bread

From Melissa Monroe McGehee's blog at Satisfyingeats.com
(Makes 10 servings; 3 grams of carbs per serving)
½ cup coconut flour
½ teaspoon baking soda
½ teaspoon baking powder
¼ teaspoon Stevia Select™ or sweetener of choice, to taste
1 teaspoon cinnamon
3 eggs
1 teaspoon vinegar
½ cup sour cream or nondairy plain yogurt
3 tablespoons salted butter or coconut oil
2 tablespoons water
(If dairy-free, add 1/8 teaspoon salt)

Preheat the oven to 350°F. Grease a loaf pan. In a medium bowl, blend dry ingredients and whisk until well combined. Add remaining ingredients and mix well. Taste for sweetness and adjust if needed. Let stand 3 minutes and then blend again.

Spread batter into loaf pan. Bake for 25–30 minutes or until a toothpick inserted into the center comes out clean. Cool on wire rack.

Strawberry/Almond Coffee Cake

(Makes 8 servings)
2½ cups almond flour
½ teaspoon baking soda
¼ teaspoon salt
¼ cup coconut oil, melted
1 tablespoon honey or maple syrup
1 teaspoon baking stevia, to taste
1 teaspoon vanilla extract
2 cups fresh organic strawberries, diced

Topping
  ½ cup almond flour
  3 tablespoons coconut oil, softened
  1 tablespoon honey or maple syrup
  1 teaspoon baking stevia, to taste
  ½–1 cup sliced almonds

Preheat the oven to 350°F. Grease an 8 8 pan with olive oil. Sift dry ingredients. Add oil, honey, stevia, and vanilla and mix with a mixer. Fold strawberries into the mix. Pour batter into the prepared pan.

Combine topping ingredients (except nuts) with a pastry cutter. Add nuts and stir until combined. Sprinkle mixture on top of the coffee cake. Bake for 25–30 minutes until a toothpick comes out clean.

LUNCH

Apple Coleslaw
  (Makes 8 servings)
  1 package coleslaw or one shredded cabbage
  1 green apple, chopped
  ½ cup walnuts, chopped
  ¼ cup green onions, diced

Dressing
  2 tablespoons olive oil
  1 tablespoon white wine vinegar
  ½ teaspoon stevia, to taste
  1/8 teaspoon salt
  1/8 teaspoon celery seeds

Place coleslaw mixture in a large salad bowl. Chop apple, green onions, and walnuts; add to coleslaw and combine. Blend dressing ingredients and pour over the salad. Combine well.

Bison Burgers

(Makes 6 servings)

2 pounds ground bison

1 bunch of scallions, chopped

¼ cup fresh parsley, finely chopped

1 teaspoon coriander

½ teaspoon cumin

1/3 teaspoon salt

¼ teaspoon pepper

¼ teaspoon cinnamon

2 tablespoons olive oil

Chop scallions and parsley. In a bowl, combine all ingredients and hand mix. Shape into thick hamburger patties. Heat oil in a skillet and cook burgers for 5–7 minutes on each side, until done.

Chicken Collard Wraps

(Makes 4 Servings)

4 large collard green leaves

3 cooked chicken thighs, diced

2 avocados, chopped

2 Roma tomatoes, chopped

4 slices cooked bacon, crumbled

Mayonnaise, to taste

Remove half of the stem from each collard leaf. Bring a pot of hot water to boil, and blanche collard leaves in boiling water for one minute. Drain and pat dry. Place collard leaves on plates. Cook 4 slices of bacon in a skillet. Chop cooked chicken, tomatoes, and avocado. Spread mayonnaise on the collard leaves. Top collards with chicken, avocado, tomatoes, and crumbled bacon. Wrap collard leaf around ingredients and hold in place with a toothpick.

Deviled Eggs

(Makes 12 servings)

12 eggs
½ cup mayonnaise
2 teaspoons of mustard
1/8 cup sweet pickles, chopped fine
¼ teaspoon salt
Paprika, for sprinkling
Pepper, dash

Place eggs in a saucepan with enough water to cover the eggs completely. On high heat bring the water to a boil. Cover and turn the heat down to low. Cook for 12 minutes. Remove from heat and rinse eggs under cold water. When eggs are cool, peel and rinse with water. Slice each egg in half lengthwise.

Remove the yolks and put them in a bowl. Mash the yolks with a fork until it is a fine crumble. Add the rest of the ingredients and stir well. Spoon yolk mixture into the well of each egg. Sprinkle with paprika.

Kale Butternut Salad

(Makes 4 servings)
1 package prewashed organic kale
1/3 butternut squash, raw, shaved slices
1 pomegranate, seeded
2/3 cup slivered almonds
½ cup roasted pepitas/pumpkin seeds

Dressing
1 lime (zest and juice)
Dash of salt
¼ cup olive oil

Place kale in a large salad bowl. Wash, peel, and shave slices of butternut squash and add to kale. Remove the seeds from the pomegranate and add the seeds to the salad. In a small bowl, zest the whole lime and squeeze juice. Add salt and oil and whisk. Pour dressing over salad and toss. Top with almonds and pumpkin seeds.

Quinoa Salad
    (Makes 6 servings)
    1½ cups quinoa, uncooked
    3 cups water
    1 cucumber, diced
    1 tomato, diced
    1 avocado, diced
    1 red bell pepper, diced
    ¼ cup green onions, chopped
    ¼ cup parsley, finely chopped
    ¼ cup mint, finely chopped

Dressing
    ¼ cup olive oil
    ¼ cup lime juice
    ¼ teaspoon white pepper
    1/8 teaspoon black pepper
    ¼ teaspoon salt

In a large pot, add water and bring it to a boil. Add the quinoa, turn down to low heat, cover and cook for 20 minutes. Allow quinoa to cool and then put it in a large salad bowl.

Chop the vegetables and herbs and add to the quinoa. In a small bowl, whisk the dressing ingredients together. Pour the dressing over the quinoa and vegetables and toss.

Sweet Potato Spinach Salad
    (Makes 6 servings)
    2 cups cooked sweet potatoes, diced
    1 green apple, diced
    ½ Vidalia onion, diced
    2 tablespoons coconut oil

1/3 teaspoon salt
¼ teaspoon cinnamon
Dash of nutmeg
2/3 cup raw pecans, chopped
1 bag of fresh prewashed spinach

Place spinach in large salad bowl. In a skillet, sauté the onion and apple in the oil for several minutes before adding the seasonings, pecans, and sweet potatoes. Cook for 1 to 2 minutes before pouring cooked ingredients over the spinach.

SNACKS/DIPS

Almond Butter

(Makes 8 servings)
2 cups raw almonds (or nuts of your choice)
Dash of salt

Preheat the oven to 325°F. Place almonds on an ungreased cookie sheet and bake for 12 minutes. Let almonds cool. If you like crunchy nut butter, take a few tablespoons of nuts out of the food processor after blending for 30–60 seconds. Set 5 tablespoons aside. Place the rest of the nuts in the food processor and mix on high for 5–7 minutes. Stop and stir the mixture about every minute. For crunchy almond butter, stir the set-aside chopped nuts into the mixture. Store in the refrigerator.

Guacamole

(Makes 8–10 servings)
5–6 avocados, smashed
½ cup cherry tomatoes, diced
2 tablespoons fresh cilantro, finely chopped
2 tablespoons olive oil
2 tablespoons red wine vinegar
½ cup chopped purple onion or scallions

    2 cloves garlic, minced (use fresh garlic, not from a jar)
    1 tablespoon lime juice

Peel and smash avocados. Chop tomatoes, onion, and cilantro. Mix all ingredients. Leave the avocado pits in the dip to preserve freshness.

Hummus
    (Makes 12 servings)
    1 cup sesame seeds
    1 clove of garlic
    2 tablespoons olive oil

Bake sesame seeds at 350°F for 20 minutes. Put roasted seeds in a food processor with garlic clove and oil. Blend until it is a smooth consistency. This is tahini. Set aside.

Dip
    4 cups dried garbanzo beans
    1 teaspoon baking soda
    3 lemons, juiced
    ½ cup lemon zest
    ½ teaspoon salt
    ½ teaspoon cumin

Soak garbanzo beans in water and 1 teaspoon baking soda overnight. Pour out the water and rinse beans. Cook garbanzo beans in water that is one inch over the top of the beans for 40 minutes or until tender. Cool and drain but set aside 1 cup of the water. Blend the beans and the rest of the ingredients in the food processor. If needed, add some of the water you set aside until the consistency of the mixture is creamy. Add the tahini and blend.

Sweet Potato Toast
    (Makes 1 serving)
    1 sweet potato

Cut sweet potato into ¼-inch diagonal slices. Pop into toaster or toaster oven and toast three different times until tender. Add toppings.

Toast Toppings
    Almond butter and honey
    Almond butter and sliced banana
    Banana and cinnamon

Trail Mix
    (Makes 8-10 serving)
    2 cups almonds
    2 cups walnuts
    2 cups pecans
    1 cup sunflower seeds
    ½ cup sesame seeds
    ¾ cup raisins
    ¾ cup craisins

Mix all ingredients together and store in a large mason jar in the refrigerator. Vary the nuts and dried fruit based on your preference. Put in resealable bags and carry with you.

VEGETABLES/SIDE DISHES

Arugula Pomegranate Salad
    (Makes 4 servings)
    1 package prewashed arugula
    1 pomegranate, seeded
    1 cup raw pecans, chopped
    Olive oil to taste
    Balsamic vinegar to taste

Place the arugula in a large salad bowl. Remove the seeds from the pomegranate and add the seeds to the salad. Add pecans, olive oil, and balsamic vinegar. Toss and serve.

Asparagus

(Makes 4 servings)
1 bunch fresh asparagus
2 tablespoons olive oil
¼ teaspoon salt

Rinse asparagus and trim bottoms. Place each asparagus single-file in a small roasting pan. Drizzle with olive oil and salt. Bake in a toaster oven at 350°F for 8–10 minutes.

Bacon Brussels Sprouts

(Makes 4–6 servings)
1 package bacon (no sugar added)
1 package fresh brussels sprouts, chopped
1/3 teaspoon salt

Cook bacon until almost done, set aside. Chop each brussels sprout into thirds and add to the bacon grease. Cook for 15–20 minutes. Chop the bacon and add to the brussels sprouts along with salt. Cook five more minutes.

Broccoli Slaw

(Makes 8 servings)
1 bag shredded broccoli or shred one head of broccoli
1 fresh pineapple, diced
1 green apple, diced
3/4 cup slivered almonds

Dressing
1 cup mayonnaise
2 tablespoons mustard
2 tablespoons white vinegar
1/8 cup stevia to taste

½ tablespoon celery seed
1 teaspoon salt
Dash of pepper

Put broccoli in a large salad bowl. Peel and chop pineapple. Chop unpeeled apple. Combine broccoli, pineapple, apple, and almonds. Whisk dressing ingredients. Pour over slaw and toss.

Coleslaw

(Makes 6 servings)
1 package shredded cabbage or shred one head of cabbage
3 grated carrots
½ cup fresh parsley, finely chopped

Dressing
1 cup mayonnaise
2 tablespoons white vinegar
Juice of one lemon
1 teaspoon salt
Pepper to taste
½ tablespoon celery seeds

Shred carrots and cabbage. Chop parsley. Combine the shredded cabbage, carrots, and parsley. In a separate bowl, whisk the dressing ingredients together. Pour over the coleslaw and toss.

Roasted Root Vegetables

(Makes 6 servings)
1 small butternut squash, chopped
1 Vidalia onion, chopped
4 carrots, chopped
1 small rutabaga, chopped
½ teaspoon of salt
Dash of pepper
3 tablespoons olive oil

Preheat the oven to 400°F. Peel butternut squash, onion, and rutabaga. Chop vegetables and place in a roasting pan. Drizzle olive oil on top and season. Roast in the oven for 45 minutes or until tender.

Roasted Carrots and Parsnips

(Makes 8 servings)
1 bag full size carrots
1 bag parsnips
3 tablespoons olive oil
2 teaspoons rosemary
¼ teaspoon salt

Preheat the oven to 400°F. Wash carrots and parsnips and trim the ends. Place in a large baking dish. Drizzle oil and seasonings on top. Bake for 45 minutes in the oven.

Slain Jane Salad

(Makes 6 servings)
2 cucumbers, diced
2 organic tomatoes, chopped
1 Vidalia onion, chopped
1 tablespoon fresh parsley, finely chopped
2 tablespoons apple cider vinegar
3 tablespoons olive oil
Dash of salt

Chop vegetables and parsley and combine them in a large salad bowl. Whisk the vinegar, oil, and salt; pour over the salad and toss.

Lillian's Sweet Potato Soufflé

(Makes 8 servings)
8 sweet potatoes
½ teaspoon Stevia Select™ or sweetener of your choice, to taste
1 tablespoon honey
½ stick butter, softened

1 cup milk or coconut milk, room temperature
1 teaspoon cinnamon
1 teaspoon nutmeg
Pinch of salt
3 egg whites
1 teaspoon baking powder
1 cup pecans, chopped

Preheat the oven to 400°F. Bake sweet potatoes in the oven for 45 minutes. Remove, cool, peel, and mash sweet potatoes. In a separate bowl, with a mixer beat the egg whites and baking powder until very stiff. With a mixer, beat the butter, stevia, and spices together, adding the sweet potatoes and milk. Fold the stiff egg whites into the sweet potato mixture. Place in a soufflé dish. Top with pecans. Turn oven down to 350°F and bake for 20 minutes.

SOUPS

Homemade Chicken Broth
(Makes 8 servings)
1 tablespoon olive oil
1 onion, chopped
2 stalks celery, chopped
2 carrots, chopped
1 whole chicken
2+ quarts of water
1 tablespoon salt
½ teaspoon pepper
1 teaspoon fresh sage

Chop vegetables and sauté in oil until onions are translucent. Add whole chicken and water and cover. Bring to a boil, then turn down heat and simmer for 2+ hours until the chicken falls off the bone. Keep adding water as needed.

Remove the chicken carcass from the broth, place on a platter, and let it cool. Pull chicken off the carcass and put it into the broth. Pour broth mixture into pint and quart mason jars. Be sure to add meat to each jar. Leave one full inch of space from the top of the jar or it will crack when it freezes as liquids expand. Place cooled jars in freezer for up to a year. Take out and use whenever you make a soup.

Homemade Vegetable Broth
(Makes 8 servings)
1 tablespoon olive oil
1 onion, chopped
2 stalks celery, chopped
2 carrots, chopped
1 head bok choy, chopped
6 cups or 1 package fresh spinach
2+ quarts of water
1 tablespoon salt
½ teaspoon pepper
1 teaspoon fresh sage

Chop and sauté vegetables in oil until onions are translucent. Add water and simmer for 1 hour. Keep adding water as needed.

Pour broth mixture into pint and quart mason jars. Leave one full inch of space from the top of the jar or it will crack when it freezes as liquids expand. Place cooled jars in freezer for up to a year. Take out and use whenever you make a soup.

Black Bean Soup
(Makes 8 servings)
1 pound dry black beans (soak in water overnight, then drain water)
1 tablespoon olive oil
2 cups onion or 1 leek, chopped
1 cup carrots, chopped
4 garlic cloves, minced
2 teaspoons cumin

¼ teaspoon red pepper flakes
4 cups chicken broth
4 cups water
¼ teaspoon thyme
2 chopped tomatoes or 1 (14 oz) can tomatoes
1½ teaspoon salt
Optional: add GF bacon or ham to flavor
Chopped green onions to garnish

Chop and sauté vegetables in oil until onions are translucent. Add the rest of the ingredients and cook on stovetop on medium-low heat for 1 hour.

White Bean and Cabbage Soup

(Makes 8 servings)
1 tablespoon olive oil
4 carrots, chopped
4 stalks of celery or 1 bok choy, chopped
1 onion, chopped
2 cloves garlic, minced
1 cabbage head, chopped
½ pound northern beans soaked in water overnight (drained)
6 cups chicken broth
3 cups water

Soak dried beans overnight in water. Drain water before cooking. Chop carrots, celery, onion, and cabbage. Sauté vegetables in oil in a large pot until mostly cooked. Add garlic and cook for 1 minute. Add the rest of the ingredients and cook on medium low heat for 30 minutes.

Brooke's Chili

(Makes 8 servings)
2 lb organic ground beef
1 diced onion

3 cloves garlic, minced
6 tomatoes, diced
1 jar tomato sauce
1 tablespoon salt
1 cup water
1 cup kidney beans (soak in water overnight, then drain)
1 cup pinto beans (soak in water overnight, then drain)
2 tablespoons chili powder
1 tablespoon cumin
1 tablespoon honey or maple syrup
1 teaspoon baking stevia
1 teaspoon pepper

In a large pot, brown the ground beef and drain the grease. Add the onion and garlic and cook until translucent. Add the rest of the ingredients and simmer for 1 hour.

Lentil Soup
(Makes 8 servings)
2 tablespoons olive oil
2 onions, chopped
1 red pepper, chopped
1 carrot, chopped
2 cloves garlic, minced
½ teaspoon cumin
¾ teaspoon thyme
1 bay leaf
8 cups chicken broth
2 chopped tomatoes
½ pound dried lentils (1¼ cup)
Optional: add GF bacon or ham to flavor
1 teaspoon salt
¼ teaspoon pepper
Handful of spinach

Chop and sauté vegetables in oil until onions are translucent. Add rest of ingredients (except spinach and spices). Cover and cook on low for 2 hours. Add spinach and spices.

White Chicken Chili

(Makes 8 servings)
1 tablespoon olive oil
1 pound of chicken strips cut into pieces
2 teaspoons cumin
½ teaspoon oregano
½ teaspoon salt
½ teaspoon pepper
1 onion, chopped
1 red bell pepper, chopped
4 cloves garlic, minced
4 cups chicken broth
2 cups northern beans (soak in water overnight, then drain)

Sauté chicken and spices in oil, then remove from pan. Chop onion and red pepper, then sauté for several minutes. Add the rest of the ingredients, including chicken, and cook on medium-low heat for 15 minutes.

Mixed Vegetable Soup

(Makes 8 servings)
1 tablespoon olive oil
1 leek, chopped
1 bok choy, chopped
4 carrots, chopped
2 cloves garlic, minced
1 zucchini, chopped
2 tomatoes, chopped
1 cup garbanzo beans (soak in water overnight, then drain)
5 potatoes, diced
8 cups broth

1 teaspoon basil
½ cup amaranth

Chop vegetables into bite-sized pieces. Sauté first four ingredients for several minutes, add garlic for one more minute. Add rest of ingredients and simmer on the stove for 25 minutes.

Potato Soup
(Makes 8 servings)
2 tablespoons olive oil
1 onion, chopped
4 cloves garlic, minced
1 teaspoon thyme
1 bay leaf
4 red potatoes, diced
6 cups water
1 leek, chopped
3 celery stalks, chopped
2 teaspoons salt
¼ teaspoon pepper

Chop vegetables into bite-sized pieces. Sauté onion, garlic, thyme, and bay leaf in oil until onions are translucent. Add rest of ingredients and simmer for about 20 minutes.

ENTREES

Chicken and Sautéed Kale
(Makes 4 servings)
5 chicken pieces, skinless
1 tablespoon olive oil
¼ teaspoon salt
1/8 teaspoon pepper
1 bunch scallions, chopped
4 dates, finely chopped

1 tablespoons red wine vinegar
½ cup homemade chicken broth
1 teaspoon rosemary

Kale
1 bunch organic kale, chopped
1 tablespoon olive oil
2 cloves garlic, minced
½ cup homemade chicken broth

Preheat the oven to 400°F. Season the chicken with salt and pepper. Heat oil in cast-iron skillet, and cook the chicken on medium high heat for 5 minutes on each side until the chicken is brown. Chop dates and scallions and add to chicken along with rest of ingredients. Transfer skillet to oven and cook for 20–25 minutes until done.

For kale, heat oil in another skillet over medium heat and add the garlic. Stir until fragrant, about a minute. Add the chopped kale and broth and stir. Cover and cook for about 5 minutes. Uncover and cook another 5 minutes until the liquid evaporated and kale is tender.

On plates, top the kale with the chicken pieces and drizzle with pan juices.

Chicken Potpie
From Melissa Monroe McGehee's blog at Satisfyingeats.com
(Makes 6 servings)
Meat & Veggie Filling
2 tablespoons of butter, ghee, or coconut oil
1 small onion, finely diced
1 red bell pepper, finely diced
1 tablespoon garlic, chopped
1½ pounds chicken meat from leftovers, diced
2 cups chicken broth, divided
½ cup cream or coconut cream
1 cup carrots, diced
1/8 teaspoon cayenne pepper

½ teaspoon salt
½ teaspoon pepper
3 to 4 tablespoons arrowroot powder

In a large frying pan over medium heat, melt butter or coconut oil, then add onion, bell pepper, and carrots. Reduce heat to medium low and add 1 1/2 cups of chicken broth and all of the cream. Add chicken, cayenne, salt, and pepper. Allow to simmer for 5 minutes on low. While simmering, make a mixture from the arrowroot powder; add ½ cup of reserved chicken stock along with 4 tablespoons of arrowroot powder to a small bowl. Whisk until powder is dissolved and there are no clumps. Pour the arrowroot mixture into the veggie and meat mixture while whisking. Taste for seasonings and adjust if needed. Cook for 1–2 minutes and then turn off the heat.

Crust
    ¾ cup plus 2 tablespoons almond flour
    1 tablespoon plus 2 teaspoons coconut flour
    1 teaspoon baking powder
    1/8 teaspoon salt
    2 tablespoons salted butter, ghee, or coconut oil, room temperature
    1 tablespoon egg white

Preheat the oven to 375°F. In a medium bowl, blend dry ingredients. Then add butter and egg white and mix with a wooden spoon until dough forms. Taste for saltiness and adjust if needed. Form dough into a ball and set aside.

For a large potpie: to ensure your dough is the correct size, on parchment or wax paper, turn the baking dish upside down and trace its shape with a pen or pencil. Place the prepared dough in the center of the marked paper. Place another sheet of parchment on top of the dough and roll out until it is the size of the marked parchment. Make sure the dough is even in thickness.

Pour prepared meat and vegetable mixture into the baking dish.

Pick up prepared crust (still on the parchment paper) and carefully invert onto meat and vegetable mixture. Carefully pull away the paper. Trim away any extra crust around the edges. Bake potpie for 35–40 minutes or until edges of the crust are slightly brown.

Fish Stew

(Makes 6 servings)
1 tablespoon olive oil
1 onion or leek, chopped
2 stalks celery, chopped
2 carrots, chopped
1 clove garlic, minced
1 tablespoon fresh parsley, finely chopped
1 bay leaf
1 clove
$1/_8$ teaspoon kelp or dulse (seaweed)
¼ teaspoon salt
Fish—leftover, cooked
2–3 cups chicken or vegetable broth

Chop the onion, celery, carrots, and parsley. Sauté vegetables in a pot on the stove until partially cooked. Add the garlic and cook for 1 minute. Add broth and seasonings. Crumble leftover fish into soup. Simmer for 20 minutes.

Lamb Butternut Stew

(Makes 6 servings)
2 pounds lamb, cubed
2 tablespoons olive oil
1 onion, chopped
2 cups water
1 small butternut squash, cubed
2-inch piece of ginger, peeled and minced
4 cloves garlic, minced
1 bay leaf

3/4 teaspoon cinnamon
½ teaspoon salt
2 firm pears, chopped

Peel and chop butternut squash. Chop onion. Peel and mince ginger. Brown the meat in oil and remove it from the pan. Add the onions and cook for five minutes on medium heat. Add the minced ginger and garlic and cook for two minutes. Add broth, butternut squash, and bay leaf. Simmer for 15 minutes. Add the chopped pears and cooked lamb. Simmer for 10 more minutes. Remove the bay leaf and serve in bowls.

Lamb Chops with Plum Sauce
(Makes 4–6 servings)
2 pounds lamb chops
3 plums, chopped
½ onion, chopped
3 cloves garlic, minced
1 teaspoon rosemary
1/3 teaspoon salt
4 tablespoons olive oil

Chop plums and onions. Heat 2 tablespoons of oil in a skillet. Add the onion and cook for five minutes. Add minced garlic and cook for one minute. Add the plums and cook for 10 minutes, stirring often. Turn off the heat and set aside.

Heat 2 tablespoons olive oil in another skillet. Sauté the lamb chops for 8 minutes on each side. Serve the chops with the plum sauce on top.

Meatballs
(Makes 6 servings)
2 pounds ground beef
½ cup fresh parsley, finely chopped
2 cloves garlic, minced

1/3 teaspoon salt

¼ teaspoon pepper

1 teaspoon red pepper flakes

1 egg

Preheat the oven to 400°F. Combine all ingredients by hand and form into 1-inch balls. Place on a cookie sheet and cook in the oven for 15–20 minutes. Serve the meatballs with a vegetable or combined with a red sauce on GF pasta or spaghetti squash.

Richard's Best Chicken

(Makes 8 servings)

2 tablespoons olive oil

8 chicken thighs, with skin on

6 cloves garlic, whole

1 16-ounce jar/can artichoke hearts, drained

¾ cup chicken broth

3 fresh squeezed oranges

1 sliced Meyer lemon

¼ cup capers

½ cup olives

Preheat the oven to 350°F. In a cast-iron skillet, fry chicken on each side in oil until the skin is golden and crispy. Remove from skillet. Sauté garlic and artichokes for a few minutes, add chicken (skin up). Pour in the rest of the ingredients and bring to a boil. Place skillet with all ingredients uncovered in the oven for 30 minutes.

Shrimp Stir-fry

(Makes 4 servings)

1 pound shrimp, raw and peeled

½ onion, diced

2 pounds green beans

1 package mushrooms, diced

4 cloves garlic, minced

2-inch piece ginger, peeled and minced
1/3 teaspoon salt
3 tablespoons olive oil

Chop onion and mushrooms. Wash and snap beans. Heat olive oil in a wok. Add all ingredients and cook for 10 minutes. Toss the ingredients often to cook evenly.

DESSERTS

Apple Coconut Cookies

(Makes 12 cookies)
4 tablespoons coconut flour
1 cup shredded unsweetened coconut
1 apple, chopped
4 pitted dates, chopped
½ teaspoon cinnamon
2 tablespoons coconut oil

Preheat the oven to 325°F. Mix all ingredients in a food processor until it makes a thick paste. Roll into 1 inch balls, then flatten cookies on a greased baking sheet. Bake in the oven for 15 minutes.

Baked Pears

(Makes 4 servings)
2 firm pears
4 teaspoons butter or coconut oil
¼ teaspoon cinnamon
1/8 teaspoon ground ginger

Preheat the oven to 350°F. Cut pears in half lengthwise and remove the core. Place on a baking pan with cut side up. Add 1 teaspoon of butter or oil on each pear. Sprinkle with cinnamon and ginger. Bake in the oven for 30 minutes.

Chocolate Brownies (Easiest and Best Ever)
From Melissa Monroe McGehee's blog at Satisfyingeats.com
(Makes 16 brownies)
1 cup GF almond or cashew butter
½ cup raw cocoa powder or unsweetened cocoa powder
½ cup sour cream or nondairy plain yogurt
2 large eggs
½ teaspoon baking soda
½ teaspoon apple cider vinegar
½ teaspoon Stevia Select™ or sweetener of choice, to taste
1 tablespoon honey (optional)
½ cup chopped pecans, walnuts, or sunflower seeds
2 tablespoons GF dark chocolate chips
Salt (optional if nut butter does not contain salt)
Extra nuts for the top

Preheat the oven to 350°F. Grease the bottom of an 8 8 square pan or 8-inch cake pan and set aside. Add all ingredients to a medium bowl, except the chocolate chips and extra nuts, and blend with mixer until smooth. Taste for sweetness and adjust as needed. Pour mixture into baking pan. Sprinkle top with chocolate chips and extra nuts. Bake for 17–20 minutes or just until the center starts to rise and hold shape. Do not overbake. Serve immediately or refrigerate for a few days to increase fudginess. These brownies taste better undercooked than overcooked.

Coconut Macaroon Cookies
(Makes 8 cookies)
3 egg whites
¼ teaspoon salt
1 teaspoon vanilla
½–1 teaspoon stevia
1½ cups unsweetened, shredded coconut

Preheat the oven to 350°F. Grease a cookie sheet. Whip the egg whites and vanilla until peaks form. Fold the rest of the ingredients into the whipped egg whites. Let the mixture stand for 5 minutes. Bake for 10–15 minutes on a greased cookie sheet until the macaroons are lightly brown.

Dark Chocolate Nut Clusters
(Makes 6–8 servings)
1 bar GF chocolate, at least 70 percent cocoa
1½ cups nuts (any variety you like)
½ cup seeds (any type)

Melt 1 bar of dark chocolate (at least 70 percent cocoa). Add a mixture of nuts and seeds until fully coated. Drop by tablespoons onto a sheet of wax paper. As the mixture cools, the nut clusters will harden. Store nut clusters at room temperature for up to one week.

Dark Chocolate Chip Pecan Cookies
(Makes 2 dozen cookies)
2 cups almond flour
1 cup coconut flour
¼ teaspoon salt
1 teaspoon baking soda
¼ cup coconut oil
1 teaspoon stevia
¼ cup maple syrup
1 egg
1 teaspoon vanilla
½ cup GF dark chocolate (more than 70 percent cocoa)
½ cup pecans, almonds, or walnuts (optional)

Preheat the oven to 375°F. Sift flours and combine dry ingredients. In a separate bowl, mix oil, stevia, syrup, eggs, and vanilla with a hand mixer. Slowly add dry ingredients. Mix by hand when adding chocolate chips and nuts. Place spoonfuls of cookie dough onto an ungreased cookie sheet. Bake for 15 minutes.

BREAD

Grace's Cornbread
   (Makes 8 servings)
   1 tablespoon olive oil for skillet
   1 cup gluten-free flour (GF flour mix)
   1 cup organic cornmeal
   4 teaspoons baking powder
   ¼ teaspoon salt
   2 eggs
   1/3 cup olive oil or butter
   ¾ cup club soda
   ¼ cup honey or stevia to taste
   1/3 cup of seeds, optional (sesame, sunflower, pumpkin)

Preheat the oven to 400°F. Heat cast-iron skillet and oil for 10 minutes in oven. In a small bowl, mix dry ingredients. In a separate bowl, whisk butter, egg, club soda, and honey. Add the dry ingredients to the wet just until mixed. Pour the seeds of your choice into the cast-iron skillet. Pour the batter on top of the seeds. Bake 15–20 minutes.

Granny Sue's Corn Pone
   (Makes 4 servings)
   ¼ teaspoon salt
   1 cup GF oatmeal
   1 cup organic cornmeal
   ¼ cup sesame seeds
   ¼ cup sunflower seeds
   ¼ cup pumpkin seeds
   1 cup hot water

Preheat the oven to 450°F. Grease a cookie sheet with olive oil. Combine all ingredients and stir. Pour ¼ of the mixture onto the prepared pan and shape like a large oval cookie about ½ inch thick. Makes four large pones. Bake for 35 minutes.

Sandwich Bread and Grain-Free Irish Soda Bread

Recipes are available from Melissa Monroe McGehee's blog at Satisfyingeats.com.

Almond Flour

Bake almonds for 15 minutes at 325°F on an ungreased cookie sheet. Let almonds cool. Place almonds in a food processor and blend on high for about 2–3 minutes until the consistency of uncooked grits. Store in a pint jar in the refrigerator or freezer. Use as a replacement for wheat flour.

APPENDIX 4: HEALTHY EATING GUIDELINES

Gluten-free, low-carbohydrate, anti-inflammatory dietary guidelines include:

- Buy organic fruits, vegetables, and meats.
- About 50 percent of your food should be fresh, organic vegetables.
- Eat one fresh, raw serving of a low-glycemic fruit per day. Low-glycemic fruits include green apples, berries, cherries, pears, plums, and grapefruit.
- Do not always eat cooked foods. Eat a couple of servings of raw vegetables every day. Eat a salad for lunch with nuts, meat, or an avocado. When eating out, order a salad or coleslaw as sides since both are raw.
- Plan for 25 percent of your food to be an animal or GF vegetable protein such as beans, nuts, and lean meats. Fish is especially nutritious.
- A variety of different raw nuts and seeds are excellent sources of protein, minerals, essential fatty acids, and naturally GF.
- Eat nontraditional grains such as quinoa and amaranth.

- Do not eat sugary cereals. Numerous GF, low-carb breakfast recipes are included in appendix 3.
- Try not to eat anything containing more than 10 grams of sugar in one serving.
- Eat cultured, GF foods such as kimchi and sauerkraut to improve gut health.

APPENDIX 5: CURB YOUR SWEET TOOTH

As you eliminate wheat, sugar, and processed foods from your diet, the craving for sugar may arise. With time your palate changes, and these cravings will be less severe. But until that occurs, the following healthy snacks will curb the sweet tooth:

- Slice a green apple, which is low in sugar, and add GF almond or cashew butter to each slice. It tastes sweet; conversely, the almond butter (recipe in appendix 3) is high in protein. Both the apple and nut butter provide fiber and fill you up.
- Melt 70-percent dark chocolate in a pan on the stove and add different types of raw nuts until well coated with the chocolate. Place mounds of nut clusters on wax paper. After an hour they harden. Keep in an airtight container on the counter or refrigerator for a week. Nuts contain fiber and are filling.
- Sparingly eat one date along with ten pecan halves. Dates are high in natural sugar, so you only need a smidgen to attain the sweetness. Don't eat too many dates, but instead fill up on the pecans, which are high in protein.

- I grow fruit trees in my yard, so from June through December I pick fresh blueberries, apples, grapes, pears, and oriental persimmons. I eat one serving of fruit each day either for breakfast or as an afternoon snack. Even if you don't have your own fruit to pick, choose organic, seasonal fruits from your grocery store or farmer's market.
- Curb sweet cravings by adding a teaspoon of raw, unfiltered, unpasteurized apple cider vinegar in a cup of water with a couple drops of stevia.

Surprisingly, taste buds change when you eat natural foods and eliminate wheat, sugar, and processed foods. It takes from a couple of weeks to months for your taste buds to stop craving sweets. With time, you will crave the nourishing foods your body needs.

NOTES

Preface
1. Maureen M. Leonard and Brintha Vasagar, "US Perspective on Gluten-Related Disorders," *Clinical and Experimental Gastroenterology*, January 24, 2014.

Introduction
1. Alessio Fasano MD, *Gluten Freedom* (Nashville: Turner Publishing Company, 2014), 32.
2. Fasano, *Gluten Freedom*, 67.

Chapter 1
1. William Davis MD, *Wheat Belly* (New York: Rodale Inc., 2011), 24.
2. Hetty C. van den Broeck, Hein C. de Jong, Elma M. J. Salentin, Liesbeth Dekking, Dirk Bosch, Rob J. Hamer, Ludovicus J. W. J. Gilissen, Ingrid M. van der Meer, and Marinus J. M. Smulders, "Presence of celiac disease epitopes in modern and old hexaploid wheat varieties: wheat breeding may have contributed to increased prevalence of celiac disease," *Theoretical and Applied Genetics* 121(8), (November 2010): 1527–39,
https://www.ncbi.nlm.nih.gov/pmc/articles/PMC2963738/.

3. Van den Broeck, et al., "Presence of celiac disease epitopes."

4. "Candida Yeast Infection, Leaky Gut, Irritable Bowel and Food Allergies," National Candida Center, https://www.nationalcandida-center.com/Leaky-Gut-and-Candida-Yeast-Infection-s/1823.htm.

5. "Candida Yeast Infection, Leaky Gut, Irritable Bowel and Food Allergies."

6. Rebecca Boyle, "How to Genetically Modify a Seed, Step By Step," *Popular Science*, January 24, 2011.

7. Leonard and Vasagar, "US Perspective on Gluten-Related Disorders."

8. Joseph A. Murray MD, *Mayo Clinic Going Gluten Free: Essential Guide to Managing Celiac Disease and Related Conditions* (New York: Time Home Entertainment Inc., 2014), 29.

9. Jonas Ludvigsson, Daniel Leffler, Julio Bai, Federico Biagi, Allessio Fasana, Peter Green, Marios Hadjivassiliou, Katri Kaukinen, Ciaran Kelly, Jonathan Leonard, Knuf Lu, Joseph Murray, David Sanders, Marjorie Walker, Fabiana and Carolina Ciacci, "The Oslo Definitions for Coeliac Disease and Related Terms," *Gut* 62(1), (January 2013): 43–52, https://www.ncbi.nlm.nih.gov/pmc/articles/PMC3440559/.

10. Fasano, *Gluten Freedom*, 32.

11. Leonard and Vasagar, "US Perspective on Gluten-Related Disorders."

Chapter 2

1. Leonard and Vasagar, "US Perspective on Gluten-Related Disorders."

2. Murray, *Mayo Clinic Going Gluten Free*, 55.

3. "Symptoms of Celiac Disease" Celiac Disease Foundation, accessed May 14, 2019, https://celiac.org/about-celiac-disease/symptoms-of-celiac-disease/.

4. Murray, *Mayo Clinic Going Gluten Free*, 111.

5. Leonard and Vasagar, "US Perspective on Gluten-Related Disorders."

6. Fasano, *Gluten Freedom*, 36.

Chapter 3
1. "What Is Celiac Disease," Celiac Disease Foundation, accessed April 10, 2019, https://celiac.org/about-celiac-disease/what-is-celiac-disease/.
2. Fasano, *Gluten Freedom,*78–79.
3. C. Catassi, Alessio Fasano, "Celiac Disease Diagnosis: Simple Rules are Better Than Complicated Algorithms," *American Journal of Medicine* 123(8), (August 2010): 6913, https://www.ncbi.nlm.nih.gov/pubmed/20670718.

Chapter 4
1. "Candida Yeast Infection, Leaky Gut, Irritable Bowel and Food Allergies," National Candida Center, https://www.nationalcandidacenter.com/Leaky-Gut-and-Candida-Yeast-Infection-s/1823.htm.
2. Julia Ross, *The Mood Cure* (New York: Penguin Group, 2002), 126.
3. Danna Korn, *Living Gluten-Free for Dummies* (Hoboken: John Wiley & Sons, Inc., 2010), 342.
4. Dale E. Bredesen, Edwin C. Amos, Jonathan Canick, Mary Ackerley, Cyrus Raji, Milan Fiala, and Jamila Ahdidan, "Reversal of cognitive decline in Alzheimer's disease," *Aging,* June 2016.

Chapter 5
1. Fran Smith, "The Addicted Brain," *National Geographic*, September 2017, 37, 43–44.

Chapter 6
1. Keri Gardner, "How Acids Affect Calcium in the Teeth & Bones," *LiveStrong*, August 14, 2017, https://www.livestrong.com/article/447824-how-acids-affect-calcium-in-the-teeth-bones/.
2. James Colquhoun, "The Truth About Calcium and Osteoporosis," *Food Matters*, November 24, 2009, http://www.foodmatters.com/article/the-truth-about-calcium-and-osteoporosis.

Chpter 7
1. Erin Schumaker, "Surgeon General Vivek Murthy: Addiction Is a

Chronic Brain Disease, Not a Moral Failing," *Huffington Post,* November 17, 2016.

2. Deane Alban, "How to Increase Dopamine Naturally," Be Brain Fit, https://bebrainfit.com/increase-dopamine/.

3. Fran Smith, "The Addicted Brain," *National Geographic*, September 2017, 36–37, 42–43.

4. Smith, "Addicted Brain," 36.

5. Davis, *Wheat Belly*, 8–9, 48–49.

INDEX

Index

ABOUT THE AUTHOR

Susan U. Neal RN, MBA, MHS, lives her life with a passion to help others improve their health. She is a Certified Health and Wellness Coach. She is the author of seven healthy living books.

- *Yoga for Beginners*
- *Scripture Yoga*
- *7 Steps to Get Off Sugar and Carbohydrates*
- *Christian Study Guide for 7 Steps to Get Off Sugar and Carbohydrates*
- *Healthy Living Journal*
- *Healthy Living Series: 3 Books in 1*

You can find Susan on SusanUNeal.com.

Health and Wellness Coaching

Do you want to improve your health? How about lose weight? Do you worry about your memory? As a Certified Health and Wellness Coach, Susan can help you move from where you are to where you want to be.

Susan will motivate you to improve your nutritional habits and hold you accountable to your goals. If you are interested, please fill out the form at Christianyoga.com/coaching.

Connect with Susan Online

Feel free to join Susan's private Facebook group at facebook.-com/7 Steps to Get Off Sugar and Carbohydrates. Through this group, she is available to answer your questions and provide you with support you may need.

Susan created the Healthy Living Series blog to provide healthy lifestyle tips and the latest scientific findings regarding foods and health. Subscribe to the blog at SusanUNeal.com/HealthyLivingBlog.

You can follow Susan on:
Facebook.com/SusanUllrichNeal
Facebook.com/ScriptureYoga/
Facebook.com/HealthyLivingSeries/
Twitter.com/SusanNealYoga
Youtube.com/c/SusanNealScriptureYoga/
Pinterest.com/SusanNealYoga/
Instagram.com/healthylivingseries/
Linkedin.com/in/susannealyoga/

Please follow Susan on BookBub and be notified when she releases a new book or when her books go on sale at Bookbub.com/authors/susan-u-neal.

SusanUNeal.com
ChristianYoga.com
SusanNeal@Bellsouth.net

OTHER PRODUCTS BY SUSAN U. NEAL

HEALTHY LIVING SERIES COURSE & BOOKS

7 Steps to Reclaim Your Health and Optimal Weight Online Course

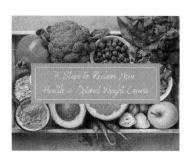

If you need additional support making this lifestyle change, purchase my course, 7 Steps to Reclaim Your Health and Optimal Weight at SusanUNeal.com/courses/7-steps-to-get-off-sugar-and-carbs-course. In this course I walk you through all the material covered in my Healthy Living Series.

I teach you the root causes of inappropriate eating habits and help you resolve those issues. One solved, taming your appetite is much easier. Learn how to change your eating habits successfully once and for all.

7 Steps to Get Off Sugar and Carbohydrates

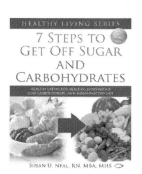

Over half of Americans live with a chronic illness and forty percent suffer from obesity, primarily due to the overconsumption of sugar and refined carbohydrates. The faith-based book, *7 Steps to Get Off Sugar and Carbohydrates* provides a day-by-day plan to wean your body off these addictive products and regain your health.

Christian Study Guide for 7 Steps to Get Off Sugar and Carbohydrates

Struggling with health problems is not our true destiny. Many of the health problems we suffer are connected to eating habits.

This study guide helps implement the plans in *7 Steps to Get Off Sugar and*

Carbohydrates. Accountability and encouragement improve your chance for success. You only have one body, and you want it to carry you through this life gracefully. Reclaim the abundant life God wants you to live. Take this journey to recover your health. You can purchase this book by clicking *Christian Study Guide for 7 Steps to Get Off Sugar and Carbohydrates.*

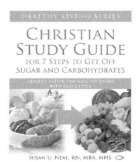

Healthy Living Journal

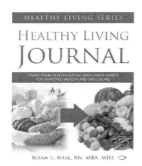

Have you tried to decrease your weight and improve your health without success? Or maybe you lost weight but gained it back. Don't allow frustration to take over. This journal will help you make and maintain healthy lifestyle changes.

During the next six weeks, commit to spend a few minutes daily recording your eating choices and how your body responds. With time you will see how different foods affect you physically and emotionally. As you record in this journal, you will begin to solve your personal health puzzle. Click here to purchase.

YOGA BOOKS

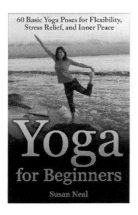

Yoga for Beginners eases you into the inner peace you long for at an easy, step-by-step beginner's pace. Through Susan's gentle encouragement, you will learn how to improve your flexibility and relieve stress. A broad range of yoga poses provides many options for the beginner- to intermediate-level student. This book includes: sixty basic yoga poses with full-page photographs and detailed explanations; three different routines to give variety; warm-up stretches; injury prevention and posture modification suggestions; and how to ease pain and anxiety.

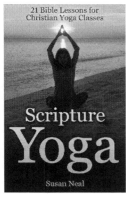

Scripture Yoga assists yoga students in creating a Christian atmosphere for their classes. Check your poses with photographs of over sixty yoga postures taken on the sugar-white sands of the Emerald Coast of Florida. A detailed description of each pose is provided with full-page photographs so postures are easily seen and replicated. You can purchase these books at ChristianYoga.com/yoga-books-decks.

HOW TO PREVENT, IMPROVE, AND REVERSE ALZHEIMER'S AND DEMENTIA

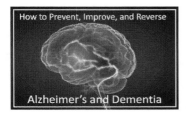

This pamphlet provides twenty-four interventions you can do to prevent, improve, or even reverse Alzheimer's and dementia. There is finally hope. To order this pamphlet go to https://gumroad.com/l/mQNTE.